FOR UPD
RECENT NEWS, &
OTHER RESOURCES ...
SEE OUR WEB SITE AT:

www.smart-publications.com

You will find:

- *A subscription offer to our free e-newsletter*

- *The latest facts and findings on the low-carb anti-aging diet*

- *A complete catalog of all our health enhancement books*

- *A directory of healthcare practitioners knowledgeable in alternative medicine*

- *Many other articles you may find of great interest and value*

SMART PUBLICATIONS™
Your Source For Alternatives

SMART GUIDE™ TO

The Low-Carb Anti-Aging Diet

John Morgenthaler
Mia Simms

SMART PUBLICATIONS™
PO Box 4667
Petaluma, CA 94955

fax: 707 763 3944
www.smart-publications.com

The Smart Guide to
The Low-Carb Anti-Aging Diet

by John Morgenthaler and Mia Simms

Published by:
Smart Publications™
PO Box 4667
Petaluma, CA 94955

fax: 707 763 3944
www.smart-publications.com

Library of Congress Catalog Card Number: 99-63894
First Printing 2000
Printed in the United States of America
First Edition

ISBN:1-890572-00-4 $9.95   Softcover

Warning - Disclaimer

Smart Publications has designed this book to provide information in regard to the subject matter covered. It is sold with the understanding that the publisher and the author(s) are not liable for the misconception or misuse of the information provided. Every effort has been made to make this book as complete and as accurate as possible. The purpose of this book is to educate. The author(s) and Smart Publications shall have neither liability nor responsibility to any person or entity with respect to any loss, damage, or injury caused or alleged to be caused directly or indirectly by the information contained in this book. The information presented herein is in no way intended as a substitute for medical counseling.

Table of Contents

Introduction

Since time immemorial, humans have searched for the Fountain of Eternal Youth. And why not? Who *doesn't* want to stay young, healthy and vibrant for a lifetime? While we may not yet know how to live forever, researchers of the past century have led us closer to the Fountain than ever.

Aging Is a Preventable Disease

Although chronological aging is a natural consequence of our physical existence, the aging process of the physical body can now be viewed as a *dis-ease* — one that may be prevented and even partially reversed. This is not merely an opinion. It is the observation of a new generation of scientists, gerontologists and life extensionists who are successfully challenging the biological process of aging.

The *Low-Carb Anti-Aging Diet* is based on cutting-edge medical research thatreveals startling information about insulin's role in aging and disease. Over the past two decades, researchers have discovered that insulin levels rise with age, and as they do, the risk of major diseases increases as well. The *Neuroendocrine Theory of Aging*, by Vladimir M. Dilman, M.D., and Ward Dean, M.D., which intricately explains the relationship between insulin and disease, describes how this ultra-potent hormone is a major factor behind many of the conditions of aging.

As you read the *Low-Carb Anti-Aging Diet*, you too, will begin to understand the significant role that insulin plays in aging and diseases such as heart disease, obesity, hypertension, type II diabetes and even cancer. You will realize how this hormone affects all of us as we age, and why the so-called middle-aged spread is often an insulin problem.

The good news is that weight gain, aging and illness caused by rising insulin levels are not inevitable. In the words of Dilman and Ward, "the main phenomena of...aging and degenerative disease are *reversible* phenomena."

It is this reversal that *The Low-Carb Anti-Aging (LCAA) Diet* addresses. Through a simple yet powerful approach to diet and lifestyle, you will learn how to control aging, shed unwanted pounds, and look and feel better than you have in years. We invite you to reach for new levels of health and well-being as you embark upon this powerful program.

Chapter 1
The Insulin-Aging Equation

One of the outstanding medical breakthroughs of the end of the last century is the discovery of insulin's role in health and disease. While many are familiar with the diabetic's relationship with insulin, few realize the critical role of this powerful hormone in their own body. It is true that insulin is essential to life; however, it tends to rise with age to levels that are too high, and, as we will see in this text, there are serious risk factors associated with elevated insulin which can hasten our demise.

The upside of this — and the topic of this book — is that insulin levels can be controlled through diet and lifestyle. It is now medically proven that optimally low levels of insulin are associated with good health and longevity. By learning how to control your insulin levels, you hold the keys to potentially slow or reverse the aging process, improve cardiovascular health, promote rapid fat loss, increase energy and mental clarity, and generate a feeling of euphoric wellness.

While the prospect of this extraordinary level of health is certainly intriguing, it is first necessary to review the role of insulin in the body.

The Role of Insulin in a Healthy Body

The amount of insulin released by the body is very simply determined by what you eat. For example, when a carbohydrate food is consumed, the process of digestion converts it into *glucose*, a simple sugar, which is absorbed into the blood stream. In response to the rise in blood sugar, insulin — sometimes referred to as the "sugar-processing hormone" — is produced by the *islets of Langerhans* within the pancreas. As insulin is released, it takes on several important functions, including the metabolism and storage of blood sugar.

Once released in response to glucose, insulin converts some of it into *glycogen*, a sugar-polymer that is stored in the liver and muscle tissues. Glycogen acts as storage fuel (like a spare gallon of gasoline for your car) and can be converted back into glucose quickly and easily on an as-needed basis. The remaining glucose circulates in the bloodstream to be used for energy. If excess glucose remains in circulation, high insulin levels will stimulate *lipogenesis* in adipose tissues (that means you're making more body fat.)

Insulin is also important for many other physiological processes. It controls appetite, acts as a growth hormone, regulates the liver's synthesis of cholesterol and signals the kidneys to retain fluid. This influential hormone also directs the flow of nutrients, such as vitamins, minerals, amino acids and fatty acids into the cells.

While these are all healthy, normal mechanisms that *should* occur, gerontologists are noticing an alarming increase in the breakdown of this metabolic process in our aging population.

Insulin and Major Diseases

Numerous studies, as well as historical and epidemiological evidence, show that consistently high levels of insulin are the primary cause of many of our nation's top killers, including several age-related disorders and diseases. For example, excess insulin is now considered a primary cause or risk factor of heart disease.[1] It is also the culprit behind the other major risk factors of heart disease, including obesity, hypertension, elevated cholesterol and triglycerides, diabetes and even certain types of cancer. [2, 3]

Insulin Resistance — When Insulin Loses Its Potency

The last several decades of medical research have identified an age-related condition known as *insulin resistance*. It is marked by the

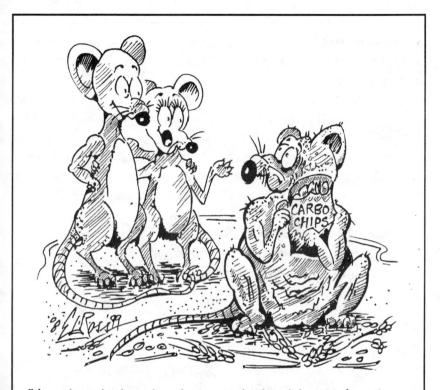

"I've decided to hook up with Freddie. He's a low-carb rat like me, and frankly he's going to live longer and healthier than you!"

gradual loss of sensitivity to insulin (the receptor sites for insulin, for whatever reason, become less responsive to insulin.) As the peripheral tissues (for example, the muscles) increasingly resist the effects of insulin, many important functions do not occur.[4]

With insulin resistance, this once powerful hormone is rendered impotent, and as a result, the entire body is negatively affected. The body responds by producing even more insulin, which results in unnaturally high levels of insulin, glucose and unabsorbed nutrients circulating in the blood stream. One of the first visible signs of the condition is weight gain, since high insulin levels hinder the conversion of glucose into energy and cause more of it to be stored as fat. Many refer to this as the "middle-age spread," not realizing that they are experiencing the early stages of insulin resistance.

Insulin Resistance and Syndrome X

As it turns out, insulin resistance is at the core of an entirely new medical disorder associated with both aging and poor lifestyle habits. Known as *syndrome X* (a term coined by a pioneer

Syndrome X is associated with a number of known risk factors for coronary heart disease

researcher, Dr. Gerald Reaven), it encompasses insulin resistance itself, along with the resulting imbalances, which often occur together in the same patient. A common but potentially deadly phenomenon, syndrome X is associated with a number of known risk factors for coronary heart disease: obesity, hypertension, elevated cholesterol and triglyceride levels, atherosclerosis, abnormal blood sugar and type II diabetes.[5,6] In addition, it is also linked with depression and mental decline.[7]

You need not have all the symptoms described above to have high insulin levels. In fact, it is even possible to be thin and have high insulin. The best way to be certain is a blood test.

Some experts estimate that as many as 50 percent of Americans may unknowingly be suffering from syndrome X. It can remain effectively hidden for years, masquerading as symptoms of other conditions. These can include fatigue, poor mental concentration, abdominal (apple-shaped) obesity, edema (fluid retention), nerve damage and an intense craving for sweets.

Still, insulin resistance and syndrome X can go undetected for up to 40 years, or until serious complications begin to surface and the pancreas just can't keep up with the demand for insulin. Some people produce two, three or four times the normal amount of insulin; yet because the cells have lost their sensitivity to the hormone, they require even more of it to maintain normal glucose levels. When the pancreas can no longer keep up, *hyperglycemia* (high blood sugar) occurs, and the diagnosis of noninsulin dependent diabetes mellitus (NIDDM or type II) diabetes often follows.

Aging and Insulin Resistance

Insulin resistance is first and foremost caused by aging. Numerous studies, including a major trial conducted by the European Group for the Study of Insulin Resistance, have determined that progressive insulin resistance is both a cause and an effect of aging.[8,9] Vladimir M. Dilman, M.D., co-author of *The Neuroendocrine Theory of Aging,* refers to insulin resistance as an "age-related pathology."[10] In other words, it is linked with the aging process of the human body.

Interestingly, the occurrences of insulin resistance and syndrome X are not exclusive to humans, and some have theorized it as a sort of "pre-programmed death." One researcher found that elevated insulin, along with increased glucose, cholesterol and triglyc-

Table 1-1

Similarity of Age-Specific Pathology and Causes of Death in Humans, Rats, and Pacific Salmon

Pathology	Man	Rat	Salmon
Insulin levels	yes	yes	?
Glucose levels	yes	yes	yes
Cholesterol	yes	yes	yes
Triglycerides	yes	yes	yes
Obesity	yes	yes	yes
Heart disease	yes	yes	yes

Source: Adapted from Waxman 1976 and Dilman 1992.

eride levels, obesity and heart disease are not only found in aging humans, but throughout a wide variety of animal species as well.[11,12] (Table 1-1)

People are often said to have died of "old age." Upon closer examination, the cause is often found to be an insulin-related problem, usually a heart attack or stroke. These conditions are so common today that to many it seems normal to develop them. With age as the primary cause of insulin resistance, this may be so; however, our modern industrialized diet does much to elicit the early onset of syndrome X.[13]

Western Lifestyle Accelerates Syndrome X

While aging is the most common cause of syndrome X, our Western lifestyle does much to accelerate its progression. Insulin resistance is hastened by a high-carbohydrate diet, and many younger people are unknowingly speeding up their own aging process by consuming excessive amounts of carbohydrates. (This applies to sugar and refined, as well as complex, carbohydrates.)[14] Diets based on carbohydrates can increase the risk of premature death, simply by increasing blood sugar levels and triggering the release of excess insulin.[15]

The human body may be designed to run on glucose as its principle fuel, but it was never meant to deal with a diet in which most of the calories are from carbohydrates as most people today consume. Other factors that contribute to syndrome X include overeating, mineral deficiencies, consumption of processed and refined foods, high alcohol intake, smoking and lack of physical exercise.[16,17,18,19] (Table 1-2)

Obesity and Insulin— Why the Fat Grow Fatter

Despite the national obsession with weight control, as a nation we are fatter today than ever. More than a third of American adults is

Table 1-2

Syndrome X Is Caused by:

- Aging
- Excessive alcohol consumption
- High carbohydrate diet
- High sugar intake
- Insulin resistance (at the core of syndrome X)
- Mineral deficiencies
- Processed foods
- Sedentary lifestyle
- Smoking

obese, yet the major cause of obesity, insulin resistance, remains largely overlooked by the medical community. Thus, it remains an unsolved mystery to those suffering from it. What is thought to be compulsivity or a behavioral problem is really an insulin predicament. That's because high insulin levels *prevent* fat loss.[20]

Lipogenesis and the Randle Effect—A Vicious Cycle

When high insulin levels prevail, *lipogenesis* (fat production and storage) is stimulated. To compound the problem, there is evidence that high insulin levels trigger the hypothalamus (the "master gland") to send out hunger signals. As a result, the insulin resistant person not only feels hungry more often, but produces and deposits fat far more readily than do healthy individuals.[21]

The dilemma can be exacerbated by what is known as the *Randle effect:* the competition between glucose and fatty acid utilization. Dilman describes it as follows: "While fats burn in the flame of carbohydrates, carbohydrates do not burn in the flame of fats."

According to Dilman, when fats and carbs are consumed together, the fats get burned as fuel, while the carbohydrates convert to glucose, and glucose converts to fat! Thus the obese, insulin-resistant person is often caught in an endless cycle of hunger, carbohydrate cravings, excessive food consumption, followed by the inevitable increase in blood sugar, insulin levels and body fat deposits. And the vicious cycle begins once again.[22]

All that increased insulin leads to increases in body fat, cholesterol, heart disease and other problems which we have described. It is a strange irony that dietary fat is usually blamed for all these things which are actually caused by the carbohydrate intake. A key point to remember, however, is that the carbohydrate intake is especially likely to cause these problems when it is consumed with dietary fat.

Obesity Begins in Childhood

Until recently, insulin resistance was thought to cause obesity only in adults, since it is considered an age-related condition. A 1998 evaluation of over 2,000 Finnish men led to the finding that insulin resistance can lead to obesity beginning in early childhood and middle age. The researchers also noted that each 5 percent weight increase, at age 20, over the average for that age, was associated with a nearly 200 percent greater risk of full-blown syndrome X by middle age.[23]

The Obesity-Osteoarthritis-Insulin Link

Obesity is often associated with osteoarthritis, a painful and often debilitating condition of the joints and underlying bone. Apparently, high insulin levels may contribute to both conditions. A recent Italian study of 48 overweight patients revealed that insulin levels were significantly higher in the obese patients who suffered osteoarthritis. Based on this and other studies, insulin resistance is now suspected as a main factor in the development of osteoarthritis in the obese.[24,25]

Insulin as Predictor of Heart Disease

Coronary heart disease is the major American epidemic of the past century, and remains the leading killer of adults in the United States. The American Heart Association estimates that one American suffers a heart attack about every 20 seconds, and every

insulin resistance can lead to obesity beginning in early childhood and middle age

minute one dies as a result. This adds up to a 1.5 million heart attacks and nearly half a million deaths every year.[26] Over the past decade, several important studies have confirmed insulin resistance as a powerful predictor of this major killer.[27]

The Finnish Helsinki Policeman study was among the first epidemiological studies demonstrating an association between high insulin levels and the risk of coronary heart disease (CHD). The trial followed 970 men between the ages of 34 to 64 years who were initially free of CHD, other cardiovascular disease or diabetes. During the 22-year follow-up, 164 men experienced a major cardiovascular event (fatal or nonfatal heart attack), which corresponded directly with the highest insulin levels.[28]

The Paris Prospective Study, which followed 7,152 men for an average of 63 months, also found a direct correlation between elevated insulin and coronary heart disease. The relationship was even more pronounced in those who were obese.[29] Another study, in *The New England Journal of Medicine,* showed that people with normal glucose tolerance but higher insulin levels were at a greater risk for coronary artery disease when compared with a group of healthy people.[30] Many, many more trials continue to demonstrate this link between insulin resistance and cardiovascular risk factors, including atherosclerotic cardiovascular disease, elevated cholesterol and triglycerides, and hypertension.[31,32,33]

Breaking News

Breathing difficulty, a common yet mysterious complication of cardiovascular disease, had researchers mystified for years. The 1998 Normative Aging Study seems to have unraveled the cause: the effects of insulin resistance on lung tissues.[34]

End Stage Syndrome X— Diabetes

Non-insulin dependent diabetes mellitus (NIDDM or type II diabetes) afflicts over 135 million people worldwide. It is the seventh leading cause of death in the United States — about every three minutes an American dies of the disease. The number of Americans with type II diabetes has tripled in the last 15 years, and it accounts for over 90 percent of all diabetic cases.[35]

Reactive hypoglycemia, hyperglycemia (pre-diabetes), and type II diabetes may all be different stages of the same condition: insulin resistance. Largely the result of diet and lifestyle, NIDDM has also been called *advanced, extreme or end stage insulin resistance,* and scientists are increasingly classifying the condition as early-onset or premature aging. Ward Dean, M.D., co-author of the *Neuroendocrine Theory of Aging,* states that "glucose tolerance gradually declines with age and by age 70 almost everyone develops some level of diabetes."

The pre-type II diabetic often produces too much insulin, which is still not enough to allow glucose into the peripheral cells. The resulting elevated glucose acts like a poison that penetrates non-insulin-dependent tissues (the lenses of the eye, nerves and arteries), causing a damaging trail of biological breakdowns. Eventually this leads to blindness, nerve damage, poor circulation, arterial damage, kidney failure, gangrene, limb amputations and ultimately a premature death.[36]

Insulin Compromises Immunity and Increases Cancer Risk

As a growth hormone, insulin is known to cause cellular division and growth. Recent studies and epidemiological evidence suggest a correlation between high insulin levels, compromised immune function and the incidence of cancer. One Danish study showed that

medical researchers are attributing long periods of elevated insulin levels to the development of certain types of cancer

high insulin levels were strongly linked with a notable decrease in the numbers of natural killer (NK) cells, lymphocytes, and monocytes, in young men.[37]

Professor Vladimir Dilman, M.D., coined the term cancerophilia to describe the increased risk of cancer associated with insulin resistance (pre-diabetes), hypothalamic insensitivity and aging. Now, medical researchers are attributing long periods of elevated insulin levels to the development of certain types of cancer, including cancers of the colon, liver, pancreas, breast and endometrium. One recent trial, which appeared in the *Journal of the National Cancer Institute*, involved 5,849 participants, 102 of whom were diagnosed with colorectal cancer. The researchers linked the incidence of this type of cancer with high insulin and glucose levels. In addition, abdominal obesity, a visible sign of insulin resistance, was also established as a risk factor of colorectal cancer. Another study showed that high insulin levels play a potential role in the growth and development of endometrial cancer.[38,39]

Aging Cannot Be Helped, but Diet Can

Insulin resistance increases with age.[40] Although our chronological clock cannot be turned back, our *biological* clock can be, at least to some degree, and is strongly influenced by what we eat. In other words, food can work for us or against us. This is actually very good news: It means that, for the most part, our life is in our hands and we can choose health and longevity. Sadly, however, most Westerners continue eating foods that do just the opposite.

Research has shown that one of the most powerful anti-aging approaches is one that controls elevated insulin levels with lifestyle modifications including the low-carb diet, regular exercise and a nutritional supplement programl.[41] Before we reveal the total solution to controlling insulin and aging, it is helpful to take a closer look at the most important controllable factor leading to insulin resistance: our Western diet.

Chapter 2
The Aging Powers of Sugar and Refined Carbohydrates

From early childhood on, our Western diet sets the stage for the perils of syndrome X. Mainly based on sugars, refined carbohydrates, oxidized and *trans*-fats (means "altered"), and processed meats, the regular consumption of these "foods" encourage insulin resistance, syndrome X, and facilitate the many disease factors that can lead us to an early grave.[42]

Our Massive Sugar Consumption

Fewer than 200 years ago, our per capita sugar consumption averaged just five pounds a year. Today, Americans eat more than 20 times that amount, at about 115 pounds of sugar per person each year. Some nutritionists unknowingly contribute to the problem by recommending a 60 percent carbohydrate diet. Once the carbs break down into glucose, they add an equivalent of about two cups of refined sugar to the bloodstream daily.[43]

> Americans eat ... about 115 pounds
> of sugar per person each year

While the human body is designed to run on glucose (blood sugar) as its principle fuel, it was never meant to deal with the constant intake of refined foods that most of us consume. Many of today's physicians and nutritionists are becoming increasingly convinced that Western dietary habits over the past 150 years are largely responsible for our prevalence of heart disease, hypertension, type II diabetes and certain types of cancer.[44]

Sugar Consumption Increases Cancer Risk

Those who consume diets high in simple carbohydrates also increase their risk of certain types of cancer. A major study of over 4,000 people compared 1,993 patients with colon and other cancers of the digestive tract with 2,410 controls. The researchers found a direct relationship between the incidence of cancer and dietary sugar consumption.[45,46]

Another study performed at a Uruguay hospital, revealed a direct link between dietary sugar intake and lung cancer. The trial, which compared 463 lung cancer patients with 465 hospitalized controls (having other conditions), evaluated the dietary patterns of these patients via a 64-item food frequency questionnaire. When the results were tallied, the researchers found that high sugar intake increased the risk of lung cancer by nearly 30 percent![47]

How Sugar Intake Leads to Premature Aging

Refined carbohydrate diets based on breads, cereals, cookies and soft drinks are now recognized as a major cause of disease and premature death.[48] With the regular consumption of these foods, the body consistently exceeds its upper limit of normal blood glucose (60 to 140 mg/dL) until it reaches a critical threshold called *hyperglycemia* (high blood sugar). The consequences of uncontrolled hyperglycemia, sometimes termed *glucotoxicity*, can be deadly for humans as well as most animal species.[49]

The most obvious effects are evident in the elderly type II diabetic, whose chronic high levels of blood sugar break down many delicate tissues, including those of the eyes, kidneys, nerves and cardiovascular system. Arshag Mooradian and Jerome Thurman, physician co-authors of *Glucotoxicity* report that "bio-

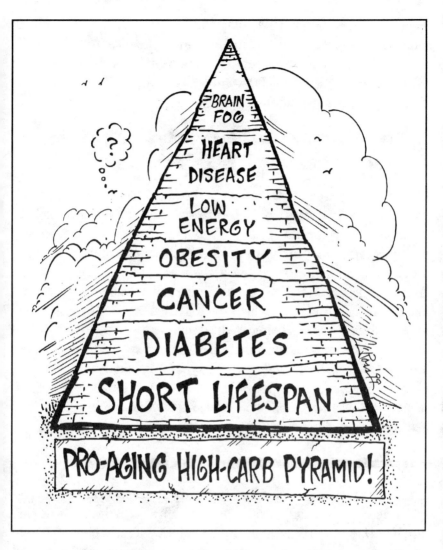

chemical and physiologic studies indicate that diabetes may be a premature-aging syndrome."[50]

Elevated Blood Sugar and All-Cause Mortality

A 20-year follow-up of three major European studies identified high blood sugar as a major risk factor for *death due to all causes.*

The European Whitehall Study, Paris Prospective Study and Helsinki Policeman Study, which combined involved over 17,000 middle-aged, nondiabetic working men, found that those who had elevated glucose levels — but were not (yet) diabetic — had a "significantly higher risk of all-cause mortality."[51]

Beware of AGEs—Advanced Glycosylation End Products

One of the significant ways in which elevated blood sugar accelerates aging may be through the formation of toxic substances called *advanced glycosylation end products* (AGEs). In the mid-1970s, biologist Anthony Cerami discovered that chronically high blood glucose is the major trigger in a chemical process that produces AGEs, which are implicated in normal and advanced aging, and age-enhanced diseases such as type II diabetes, atherosclerosis, kidney disease and Alzheimer's disease.[52]

AGEs form at accelerated rates whenever blood-sugar levels are high. This is most evident in the type II diabetics, who, in their chronic state of hyperglycemia, produce far more AGEs than healthy people do. Recent studies also show that sunlight exposure can further accelerate AGEs-related damage.[53]

AGEs and Cross-Linking

The production of AGEs, which normally increases with age, eventually leads to damaging responses within the body, such as the *cross-linking* of collagen. Sometimes referred to as a carmelization or browning reaction, this particular type of cross-linking involves a chemical reaction between sugar and protein molecules that inflicts serious damage to cell membranes and collagen fibers. Eventually this cross-linking leads to the stiffening of connective tissue.[54]

As cross-links increasingly reduce the flexibility and permeability of tissues and cells, cellular communications and repair processes also begin to break down. With time, the tissues of the body become irreversibly transformed, and aging, disease and death finally gain the upper hand.

As bleak as this sounds, this type of cross-linking can be slowed through blood-sugar and insulin control.

Control Aging Through Good Glycemic Control

Remember, AGEs production and glucose-related cross-linking happen the fastest when blood sugar levels are chronically high. This means that good blood-sugar control is absolutely essential for anti-aging and disease prevention.[55] In this book, we'll offer two highly effective ways to do this:

The Low-Glycemic-Index (LGI) Diet.

The Low-Carb Anti-Aging (LCAA) Diet.

Chapter 3
The Low-Glycemic Index Diet

As presented in the previous Chapter, the food we eat very literally affects the development and progression of health and disease in the body. One solution to the predicaments of insulin resistance and high blood-sugar levels begins with a fairly recent development in food evaluation called the *glycemic index* (GI).

The glycemic index is a rating system that can help you make food choices that lead to a slower, more gradual conversion of carbohydrates into glucose and therefore a lower, slower release of insulin. This resulting improvement in glycemic and insulin control can decrease body fat, improve energy levels, reduce serum cholesterol, prevent and reverse hypertension and improve cardiovascular health. Good glycemic control can also reduce toxic AGEs, the cross-linking of collagen and free radical damage.[56,57,58]

How Foods Are Rated on the Index

Although it is not an exact science, the glycemic index indicates the effect a particular food has on blood-sugar levels. It is the result of years of study and volumes of exhaustive research by many researchers. Here's how it works: All foods are assigned a numerical value ranging from 0 to 150, which is actually a gauge of blood sugar response to common foods and beverages in healthy volunteers. The compilation of these is now referred to as the glycemic index.

It is important to note that there are two approaches to the glycemic index. One is based on white bread having an assigned value of 100, the other is based on glucose having an assigned value of 100. With white bread as the standard, other foods are gauged relative to it. For example, white spaghetti would receive a rating of 67. If glucose is the standard, the spaghetti receives a rating of 50, meaning it produces half the rise in blood sugar as glucose (see table 3-1).

Table 3-1

Comparisons of the Two Standards of Glycemic Index

Food (50 grams)	Index 1*	Index 2**
Glucose	138	100
White bread	100	72
White spaghetti	67	50

* Index 1: white bread as the standard
** Index 2: glucose as the standard

High Glycemic vs. Low Glycemic Foods

High glycemic index foods such as a piece of white bread cause a rapid breakdown and conversion of carbohydrate into glucose and therefore a rapid rise in blood sugar. These foods are rated as "high glycemic" on the index. They are not good food choices for anyone, as they jolt the pancreas into releasing sharp, shocking amounts of insulin. Conversely, foods such as pinto beans (see table x), that promote a slower, sustained release of glucose and insulin are considered as having a "low glycemic" rating. This is the basis of the Low Glycemic Index (LGI) Diet.[59,60]

Obesity Begins with High Glycemic Foods

Researchers are finding that obesity, which usually begins in childhood, is strongly related to the consumption of high glycemic foods. One study of obese teen-age boys demonstrated how high glycemic foods lead to patterns of binging and obesity. The teens were offered various glycemic foods and evaluated based on their response to them.

When compared with low GI foods, high GI foods caused rapid glucose absorption, higher blood sugar, insulin and fatty acid levels, and an increase of adrenaline. After eating the high glycemic index foods, the boys also resorted to binge-type eating behavior, which was most likely due to insulin spikes (which stimulates appetite) and adrenal stimulation![61]

High Glycemic Foods Increase Cancer Risk

A recent Italian survey showed that the consumption of high-glycemic foods may lead to an increased risk of cancer. The diets of 1,953 cancer patients were compared with 4,154 hospitalized controls suffering from unrelated conditions. All of the patients were interviewed using a 79-subject questionnaire, complete with food lists and recipe ingredients. The results revealed a remarkable trend: The cancer patients were those who consumed the highest percentage of high-glycemic foods, which included refined breads, sugars, cereals, potatoes, cakes and candies. The researchers concluded that the high-glycemic foods lead to insulin resistance and the resulting development of cancer.[62]

The same survey showed that fish, vegetables and fruits had a negative association with cancer risk. And butter, eggs and flesh foods, including white, red, and processed meats, seemed noninfluential.[63]

Caution—Some "Health" Foods Are Not So Healthy!

It might seem that all refined carbohydrate foods have a high glycemic index, while all complex carbohydrate foods have a low glycemic index. But this is not always the case. Take a look at Table 3-2 and notice how some vegetables and grains such as carrots, potatoes and rice exhibit a surprisingly high GI! These foods produce a more rapid rise in blood glucose than table sugar! Equally unexpected is the fact that some simple sugars such as fructose have a lower glycemic index than many vegetables, grains and legumes (see Table 3-2).

• •

Important Note: Fructose should be used only with moderation. While fructose does have a low glycemic rating, it can still produce insulin resistance, increase triglycerides, and promote fat storage. As revealed by a 1998 study in the *Journal of Nutrition*, the long-term consumption of fructose can also produce several pro-aging effects, including the increased production of AGEs (see Chapter 2).[64]

• •

Low Glycemic Index Diet Reverses Syndrome X

As the Low Glycemic Index Diet helps to control blood sugar and insulin levels, it simultaneously reduces the risk of premature aging and disease and can enhance overall health and well-being. In fact, the consistent consumption of low glycemic foods has been shown to improve health, reduce body fat, sustain energy levels, heighten mental clarity and prevent the cardiovascular risk factors known as syndrome X.[65]

Good Glycemic Control Reduces Free-Radical Damage

Good glycemic control can significantly reduce free-radical damage and delay the onset of advanced glycosylation end products (AGEs — see Chapter 2).[66] In this way, the LGI Diet is especially helpful for the diabetic, as it can help reduce chronically elevated blood values down to safer values.*

Choose Fresh, Wholesome Low Glycemic Foods

The LGI Diet emphasizes the consumption of foods with a glycemic rating of about 60 or lower (on the glucose-standard system). This includes foods such as pasta, plain yogurt, chick peas, pinto beans, peanuts, apples, strawberries and whole grain rye bread (see table 3-2).

The LGI Diet emphasizes the consumption of foods with a glycemic rating of about 60 or lower

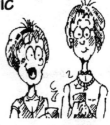

Some of the best food choices, however, are not even listed on the glycemic index chart. That's because they have such a naturally low rating that researchers don't even bother to test or list them. They include the non-starchy vegetables, such as leafy greens, celery, broccoli, cauliflower, zucchini, avocado, tomatoes, sprouts and jicama (for more examples, see Chapter 4, shopping list). These have a glycemic rating below 20, are rich in nutrients and enzymes, and should be the cornerstone of any health-promoting anti-aging program.

---

* The glycemic index was originally developed to help diabetics make better food choices.

Protein-rich foods like meat and fat-rich food like vegetable oils do not contain enough carbohydrates to be of concern — they are excellent food choices. Choose hormone- and antibiotic-free

Table 3-2

Glycemic Index of Selected Foods*

Using Glucose as the Standard of Comparison

Food	GI
Glucose	100
Potato, baked	98
Carrots, cooked	92
Honey	92
White rice, instant	91
Cornflakes	84
Honey	74
Bread, white	72
Bagels	72
Potatoes, mashed	70
Bread, wheat	69
Table sugar	65
Beets	64
Raisins	61
Oatmeal	61
Bran muffin	60
Pita	57
Popcorn	55
Buckwheat	54
Banana	53
Potato chips	51
Green peas	51
Ice cream	50
All-bran cereal	44
Whole-grain rye bread	42

Pinto beans	42
Pasta	41
Apples	39
Tomatoes	38
Yogurt, plain	38
Chick peas	36
Skim milk	32
Strawberries	32
Kidney beans	29
Peaches	26
Cherries	24
Fructose	20
Soybeans	15
Peanuts	13

*Note: Non-starchy vegetables such as leafy greens (lettuce, spinach, kale), sprouts, and broccoli are not listed due to their extremely low rating. Meat, poultry, fish, eggs, cream, fats and oils, which are extremely low carbohydrate foods, are not rated.

meats and poultry, as well as omega-3-rich coldwater fish (see Chapter 7). Soy foods such as tofu, soy flour and texturized vegetable protein (TVP) are also excellent choices. (Remember to check food product labels to confirm exact carbohydrate amounts.)

Menu Suggestions

Breakfasts

- Cottage cheese with half a cup strawberries, sprinkled with whey protein concentrate (see Chapter 6), slivered almonds and cinnamon

- Whole-grain rye toast with one or two poached eggs

- Old fashioned oatmeal mixed with vanilla whey protein concentrate

- Non-fat plain yogurt with blueberries, sweetened with stevia
- All-bran cereal with unsweetened soy milk and sliced peaches

Lunches

- Steamed vegetable platter with black, kidney or pinto beans, topped with grated cheddar cheese
- Chicken-vegetable soup with buttered whole-grain rye toast and tomato slices
- Vegetarian lasagna with a vegetable salad topped with chickpeas
- Turkey burger with onions and sprouts stuffed into a half toasted pita bread
- Warmed corn tortilla topped with refried beans, shredded lettuce, onion, tomato and cheese

Dinners

- Chicken vegetable stir-fry with kasha (buckwheat groats)
- Scallops sautéed in butter and garlic with steamed vegetables
- Sushi with seasoned green soybeans and miso soup
- Spinach ravioli with tomato sauce. Tossed green salad with dressing
- London broil, grilled vegetables and one slice whole-grain rye bread

Desserts or Snacks

- Stevia-sweetened plain yogurt with fresh cherries
- Low glycemic protein shake
- Bran muffin
- Vegetables slices with bean dip
- Handful of peanuts or almonds

Get the Sugars Out
with Herbal Stevia rebaudiana

Stevia rebaudiana is a herbal sweetener native to Paraguay and Brazil, where it has been used as a sweetener for over 1,500 years. In the early 1970s a group of Japanese companies developed a method of extracting the sweet *steviosides* from the stevia leaf to produce a fine white powder that is about 300 times sweeter than table sugar.

One teaspoon of finely ground stevioside is equivalent to about one cup of sugar. It is also calorie-free, does not raise blood glucose levels and boasts a number of other therapeutic benefits. Considering the negative effects of sugar and artificial sweeteners, we recommend stevia as a healthy sweetening alternative.[67]

The Choice Is Yours

Once you become familiar with the high glycemic foods to avoid, this diet becomes relatively simple to follow. By cutting out high-glycemic carbohydrates and emphasizing wholesome low-glycemic foods such as non-starchy vegetables, low glycemic fruits, selected whole grains, and healthy proteins and fats, good results can be achieved.

While the Low-Carb Anti-Aging (LCAA) Diet will yield faster results (see Chapter 4), the Low Glycemic Index (LGI) Diet is designed for those who want to control insulin and blood sugar, yet still feel the need to consume some carbohydrates. However, if cravings, weight gain or binge-patterns prevail, the LCAA Diet may be more appropriate for you.

To ensure the consumption of low-glycemic foods only, we recommend that you purchase a complete glycemic index counter or contact the Glycemic Research Institute.* You can also check the Smart Publications website (at www.smart-publications.com) for the latest updates in this area. Be sure to subscribe to the free e-newsletter while you're there.

Hot Tip: Use stevia as a natural, non-caloric sweetener.

Website: Please check our website at www.smart-publications.com. You will find information on how to order nutritional products by mail (for better selection and to save money), pointers on finding a suitable physician and a subscription button for our free e-newsletter.

Sources: For more information on the glycemic index of foods, contact the Glycemic Research Institute at 601 Pennsylvania Ave., N.W., Washington, D.C. 20004; telephone: (202) 434-8270.

Chapter 4
The Low-Carb Anti-Aging (LCAA) Diet

S ome life extensionists are taking the low glycemic anti-aging approach to an extreme — with excellent results. It's called the Low-Carb Anti-Aging (LCAA) Diet and can reduce elevated insulin levels, balance blood sugar, produce rapid fat loss, profoundly enhance mental clarity, improve muscle tone, reduce serum cholesterol, lower blood pressure and promote a longer, healthier life. Assuming that ideal health, body weight and maximum life span are your priorities, the LCAA Diet offers an approach that is unparalleled in its effectiveness.

The Low-Carb Anti-Aging Diet has all the benefits of the Low-Glycemic Index Diet, yet is designed for accelerated weight loss and more effective reversal of the conditions associated with insulin resistance (syndrome X). As a very low-carbohydrate program, it is unique in that it also emphasizes nutrient-rich foods with age-reversing, disease-defying and immune-enhancing properties (see table 4-1).

Carbohydrates Are Not a Required Nutrient

When people learn that the LCAA Diet requires a drastic reduction of carbohydrates, they sometimes express a combination of shock, confusion and disbelief. After all, aren't carbohydrates considered the fuel of life? Aren't carbohydrates the very foundation of our metabolic system? In some ways, carbohydrates are. But they are also non-essential.

Table 4-1

Benefits of the LCAA Diet

- Balanced Blood Sugar
- Better Muscle Tone
- Enhanced Well Being
- Improved Immunity
- Increased Longevity
- Lower Cholesterol and Triglyceride Levels
- Mental Clarity
- No Hunger
- Optimally Low Insulin Levels
- Reduced Blood Pressure
- Reduced Body Fat
- Safe, Rapid Weight Loss

Our bodies like carbohydrate because it is convenient, quick and plentiful during the season immediately before winter. Carbohydrates help us lay down fat for the coming winter when food will be scarce. While winter food may have been scarce during paleolithic times, it is no longer so. We have access to fresh produce almost year round and no longer need to get fat to survive.

To better understand this, it is helpful to review the three *macronutrients* of food: proteins, fats and carbohydrates. While all three are capable of providing energy to the body (being burned for calories), proteins and fats are used extensively for structural purposes. Extensive amounts of proteins and fats are required for tissue growth, maintenance and repair. Only traces of carbohydrates are required for these purposes. The primary function of carbohydrate is energy production, and this function can be substituted by fat and protein. In other words, carbohydrate is basically non-essential. Of the three macronutrients, the body can live without only one: carbohydrates.

The role that carbohydrate plays in energy production depends on the availability of carbohydrate in the diet. When carbohydrate is present, the body burns it preferentially. When carbo-hydrate is limited, the body turns to fat as its primary energy source. When carbohydrate is restored, the body shuts down fat-burning systems and opens up carbohydrate energy pathways.

Eat fat to get lean and eat carbohydrate to get fat!

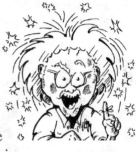

When carbohydrate is present in excess, the body converts it to fat. This process, called lipogenesis or fat neogenesis, is activated whenever carbohydrate intake exceeds carbohydrate energy needs. This process is the reason that carbohydrate-rich diets make people fat.

Eat fat to get lean and eat carbohydrate to get fat. While this may seem double counterintuitive at first blush, this is the reality of our biochemistries. Human ancestors who were not efficient at con-verting the carbohydrate-rich harvest of the summer into fat were doomed to starve during the following winter. Those ancestors who could efficiently convert carbohydrate into fat survived. We are the progeny of those ancestors.

The eat-fat-to-get-lean part of the equation is equally difficult to understand, given the extensive advertising of food suppliers selling fat-free this and low-fat that which imply that avoiding fat is the quickest way to get lean. But metabolism doesn't necessarily work that way. If you eat fat "with" carbohydrate, the fat-burning pathways remain inactive. But if you eat fat without carbohydrate, fat-burning pathways are open and can burn up all the fat, making you lean. This is the essential concept behind the LCAA diet: keep the fat-burning pathways open!

Protein Requires Energy to Be Metabolized

When the body uses carbohydrates for fuel, it readily converts them into glucose. This is a relatively simple process and utilizes very little energy. However, when the body resorts to using protein for fuel, it requires a great deal more energy to digest and metabolize that protein in order to convert it into glucose. In fact, it takes 47 percent more energy to digest and metabolize proteins than carbohydrates, which explains why protein foods minimally affect insulin levels.[68]

Only Carbs Significantly Affect Insulin

Because carbohydrates readily convert to glucose, they have a significant effect on insulin levels. Fats consumed alone have no affect on insulin. Proteins consumed alone have a minimal effect on insulin. Carbohydrates, therefore, are the *only* macronutrient that significantly affects our insulin levels.

The Basics of the LCAA Diet

With the understanding that high insulin levels are at the core of syndrome X and other diseases of aging, and the knowledge that carbohydrates (which increase insulin levels) are not a dietary requirement, we have created the LCAA Diet as an anti-aging program that restores insulin and blood sugar levels by drastically reducing the intake of carbohydrates.

LCAA Diet foods include healthy proteins, fats and low starch vegetables that do not cause sharp rises in insulin. This approach to eating allows the following changes to occur:

- Burning off of excess glycogen stores.
- Accessing alternative fuel sources, including protein and fat, and *the body's own fat* (ketosis).
- Reversing of hyperglycemia (high blood sugar), hyperinsulinism (elevated insulin levels), insulin resistance, premature aging and syndrome X.
- Rapid weight loss, fat loss, mental clarity and physical well-being.

The LCAA Diet effects these changes by encouraging the body to enter a fat-burning state called *ketosis*.

A Word About Fruit

Some unprocessed carbohydrate foods can be safely consumed with the LCAA diet, providing that the amount is less than what can be immediately burned through exercise. So, if you want to eat an apple (low glycemic) or a handful of grapes (high glycemic), all you have to do is increase your activity level to burn off the extra calories. This principle can be applied to most situations where you might eat too much carbohydrate due to eating out, dining with family or friends (holiday meals) or indulging a craving ("falling off the wagon").

The LCAA Ketosis Diet — Restoring Insulin and Glucose Balance

The LCAA Diet is designed to produce a state of dietary ketosis, which has an exceptionally rejuvenating effect on the body. Being in ketosis is the quickest, safest way to control blood sugar and hyperinsulinism, while simultaneously burning off excess body fat. The key to the diet's effectiveness is a shift in the body's fuel supply. When carbohydrate intake is sufficiently lowered, the metabolism shifts from a glucose-based energy supply to one that utilizes the body's own fat. This fat-burning mechanism occurs during sleep, fasting and when insulin levels are low. [69]

After 48 hours with virtually no carbohydrates, the absence of glucose induces lower insulin levels, which causes the desired metabolic shift. As the body enters into lipolysis, ketosis is achieved. First, fat tissues (triglycerides) are split into glycerol and free fatty acids. These are broken down into simple compounds called *ketone bodies*, which in turn are used as fuel by the brain and muscles. According to the research of Robert C. Atkins, M.D., pioneer and original crusader for the low carbohydrate diet, *the brain tissues utilize these ketone bodies more readily than glucose* and in fact prefer them as a fuel source.[70]

How to Achieve Ketosis

Ketosis is achieved by reducing carbohydrate intake below a threshold. Since this threshold can be significantly different from person to person, many people eliminate practically all carbohydrate to accelerate the process. By eating only healthy meats (or tofu) and low-carbohydrate vegetables, the metabolic switch over takes place as swiftly as possible. When the body enters ketosis, ketones are released into the blood stream and urine, where that can be detected with urine test strips. A positive urine test for ketones is proof that the body has entered ketosis and it is chemical evidence that adipose tissue or stored fat is being burned.

A Measure of Success

To determine the degree of ketosis, special testing strips are available over-the-counter (OTC) at pharmacies. They may be purchased as either Lipostix® or Ketostix®.

To ensure that ketosis has been reached, a testing strip may be dipped into a sample of urine at the end of the second day or touched to the stream of urine while urinating, if that is more convenient. Ketosis is indicated by a change in the color of the strip. A slight state of ketosis is reflected by a light pink color with dark redish-brownish-purple indicating an extreme state of ketosis. Although fat burning may be maximized by extreme ketosis, don't try to stay in that state. Extreme ketosis may cause high levels of beta-ketobutyrate to accumulate, which can spontaneously break down into acetone. Acetone is fairly toxic and is not efficiently metabolized, so it is eliminated by outgassing through the lungs, imparting a solvent smell to the breath. It is best to avoid this possibility by keeping ketosis to low and moderate levels.

It is also worth mentioning that your body can be actively metabolizing fat (through beta-oxidation) without being in ketosis. If you are on a low-carbohydrate diet yet not in ketosis but you

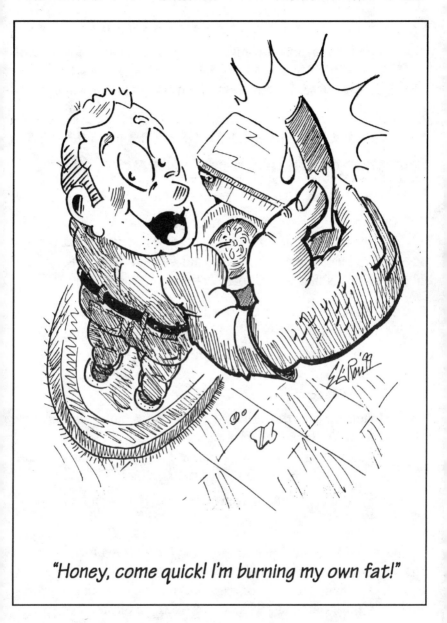

"Honey, come quick! I'm burning my own fat!"

body fat percentage is going down and your energy level is good, there is not necessarily a need to be in ketosis. Another way to say this is: Treat your body, not the test strips. If you are getting the right results and you feel good, that is what we're after.

● ●

Hot Tip: Insufficient water intake can cause concentrated urine and *the false impression of elevated ketones.* Therefore, it is important to drink plenty of water when following this diet.

● ●

Dietary Guidelines—Ready, Set, Go!

To reduce body fat and turn back the biological clock as quickly as possible, begin by scheduling a health assessment with a trusted physician, clearing the refrigerator and cupboards and restocking them with foods that will restore health.

Ready—Schedule an Overall Health Assessment

• Inform your physician that you would like to start this diet. Certain medications, such as anti-diabetes drugs and insulin, can be dangerous on this diet.

• Make sure your health evaluation includes blood tests of cholesterol, triglycerides, blood glucose and fasting insulin levels, as well as a test of uric acid levels. Test results should change for the better as you follow this diet.

• Ask for a complete thyroid panel and glucose-tolerance test before beginning this diet.

Important Note: Before initiating this or any other diet program, it is best to do so under the guidance and knowledge of a trusted physician. If you are pregnant, nursing or taking medications to control blood sugar, blood pressure, cholesterol or edema (fluid retention), this is particularly important.

Set—Clear the Cupboards

It is best to begin the LCAA Diet feeling prepared. Following are some suggestions that will help:

- Clear the refrigerator and cupboards of all sugar and carbo-hydrate-containing products. Restock them with plenty of foods that you like (see the shopping list at the end of this Chapter).

- Abstain from any non-essential drugs, including over-the-counter medications such as cough syrups and drops. Also eliminate or drastically reduce the use of alcohol (spirits, wine and beer) and any other recreational drugs. **Remember: This is an anti-aging program.**

- Procure a carbohydrate gram counter, available at most book-stores, or check the Smart Publications web site (at www.smart-publications.com).

- Document your "before" state with photos, weight measure-ments, body-fat percentage and body dimensions. The more the merrier. You might even use your home video camera to make a time-lapse video of your body changes.

GO!—Get into Ketosis

The following guidelines help you achieve and maintain ketosis as quickly as possible:

- For the first two or three days, or until ketosis is achieved, eat only meat, fish, poultry, tofu, zero-carbohydrate protein pow-ders, eggs, cheese, cream, fats and oils. In addition, one or two dinner salads may be consumed, for a **maximum of 10 to 20 carbohydrates** per day.

- Once in ketosis, you can increase your carbohydrate intake somewhat. Just keep checking your ketosis level with the urine test strips described above and eat only so much carbo-hydrate such that you stay in a state of mild ketosis. For some people this means no more than **30 carbohydrates** a day, other people can get away with much more and still be in mild ketosis. Carbohydrate foods should consist of leafy greens and other low-carbohydrate vegetables (see shopping list at the end of this Chapter) and should be **organically grown** whenever possible.

 Important Note: Some protein foods such as eggs, tofu, dairy, soy and whey protein concentrate contain trace amounts of carbohydrates. Check labels and/or your carbohydrate counter.

- Choose wholesome, minimally processed **protein** sources. Look for organic or free-range meats, poultry, eggs and dairy products.

- Choose pure, unprocessed **fats and oils**, organically grown and cold-pressed whenever possible:

    Stick with healthy fats (see Chapter 7).

    Mayonnaise is also recommended (check label for carbohydrates).

    All oils that are liquid at room temperature should be refrigerated to avoid rancidity.

    Coconut oil and coconut milk may help promote ketosis and encourage healthy thyroid function.

    Do not buy or consume any food that has the words "partially hydrogenated" on the label. This includes such obvious products as margarine and may include peanut butter, baked goods, processed oils and more.

    Do not use Olestra.

    Avoid consumption of rancid (oxidized) fats. This may include aged or improperly preserved vegetable oils (especially the more highly polyunsaturated oils) and dietary supplements containing vegetable or fish oils. Peroxidized fats impart "off" flavors (acrid, bitter tastes) to these products, but the taste threshold for rancidity is pretty high (you can miss it at the early stages of rancidity). If you can taste it, you should have thrown it out a week earlier.

- Consume about 25 grams of **fiber** each day. The best way to do this is by eating plenty of vegetables and, if necessary, using a psyllium husk fiber supplement (no sugar added).

- Eat more frequently than you might otherwise. Space meal about four to five hours apart, inserting low-carb snacks or extra meals to make this work.

- Spread out your limited carbohydrate intake throughout the day. Try to engage in some form of exercise after any above-ideal carbohydrate intake or alcohol use. Walking is a good option. If you go out to drink, use the dance floor to work off the alcohol.

- Eat when hungry and to satiation, but **never overeat** or gorge yourself.

- Take a quality, high-potency **vitamin-mineral** supplement (see Chapter 8).

- Drink at least eight 8-ounce glasses of **purified water** every day (see Chapter 8).

- Write down your **goals** and post them where you'll see them often (the bathroom mirror).

- **Reread these guidelines** frequently — and more important-ly, stick with them!

How to Kick Start Ketosis

Although the carbohydrate restriction described above will shift your body into ketosis, the shift into ketosis can be made more quickly and effortlessly if enhanced by the following extras:

- Coconut oil — two to four tablespoons per day (this if for the medium chain triglyceride, MCT, content),

- CoQ10 – 150mg per day

- Carnitine (or acetyl-l-carnitine) — 1500-3000mg per day

- Exercise — daily

These nutrients (plus the exercise) function as a mitochondrial support and stimulant program and will make the shift into ketosis smooth and effortless. There is so much more we could say about nutritional support of mitochondrial function. In fact, this protocol (coconut oil, CoQ10, carnitine and exercise) could be a whole book in itself. However, the topic is far outside the scope of this effort so we'll have to leave for now.

Beware of Carbohydrate Addiction

When you cut out carbohydrates, you may discover that you are addicted. Carbohydrate withdrawal is often experienced as a gripping craving for carbohydrate-rich foods (including sweets or alcohol). In Western diets, carbohydrate addiction is probably a lot more common than most people realize. Carbohydrate withdrawal is most severe in the first few days of the LCAA diet, before ketosis kicks in.

After day three, carbohydrate cravings usually subside greatly. You may want to re-read this section several times to remind yourself that it will go away if you persevere. Tell yourself that a few days of discomfort are worth the long-term reward of a healthier life without carbohydrate compulsions.

By the time ketosis is achieved, you will be grateful you stuck it out. You will notice that, almost as if by magic, sugar and carbohydrate cravings have virtually disappeared. In their place you will most likely feel a wonderful sense of clarity, newfound energy and well being.

What Foods Contain Carbohydrates?

- Bread, pasta, crackers, flour, potatoes, carrots, peas, corn, fruits, baked goods, candies, chewing gum, sugars.

- All dairy foods, except whey protein concentrate, butter,

cream and cheeses. Cultured milk products like cheese, cottage cheese and yogurt have dramatically reduced carbohydrate and increased protein content.

- Some medications, including cough lozenges and syrups.

- Imitation crab, shrimp and lobster meat. These often contain starch and sugar.

- All fruits contain simple sugars/carbohydrates. Most berries, however, are both low glycemic and low in carbohydrates. Once in ketosis, strawberries, blueberries and raspberries may be eaten in small amounts.

• •

Caution: A single "innocent bite" of a carbohydrate food can set you back considerably. Remember your goals and choose your food and beverage selections wisely.

• •

Beware of Hidden Carbohydrate Sources

A number of foods that appear to be low-carb, yet are often laden with hidden sugars and starches. The following are the most common sources:

- **"Sugar-free" products**, such as gum, breath mints and cough drops. Many of these contain non-sucrose sweeteners that contain carbohydrates: sorbitol, mannitol, maltose, fructose.

- **Salad dressings and condiments**, including mayonnaise (some brands), ketchup, relish and pickles. Check the labels for sugar and carbohydrate content.

- **Gravies and sauces**: These usually include starches as thickeners, sweeteners or flavor enhancers.

- **Dairy products:** yogurt, milk, half-and-half, diet cheeses and cheese spreads all contain carbohydrates.

- **Restaurant foods:** Flour or bread crumbs are usually used for sautéeing meat, fish or poultry.

- **Alcohol:** Any alcohol-containing beverage. Alcohol acts like a powerful carbohydrate on energy pathways, rapidly shutting down fat-burning pathways.

Avoid These Unhealthy Low-Carb Foods

The following foods may be low-carb. However, they are sources of health-damaging fats, chemicals, additives, preservatives, sugars and/or starches:

Processed meats, processed and imitation cheeses (American cheese), margarine, shortening (Crisco), artificial sweeteners, non-dairy creamer, Olestra and other synthetic foods. **Avoid them!**

• •

 A Final Caution: Never assume a food is low-carbohydrate. Read the label and check your carbohydrate counter.

• •

Menu Suggestions

Breakfasts

- Smoothies (low-carb "shake") made with a quality whey protein concentrate and/or soy protein powder. These may be fortified with vitamins and minerals (check carbohydrate count).

- Eggs or an egg dish: scrambled, poached, soft boiled or omelet with vegetables and cheese.

- Crunchy lettuce leaves topped with lox, cucumber slices and cream cheese. Sprinkle with pepper and paprika.

- Pancakes made from low-carb mix (see Resources), topped with sour cream and sprinkled with cinnamon.

Lunch

- Broiled chicken with a salad and creamy dressing.

- Grilled hamburger patty with lettuce, tomato slices, cheese, mayonnaise and mustard.

- Tuna, chicken, egg or tofu salad over a bed of baby lettuce with minced chives.

- Thai chicken-coconut soup with mung bean sprout salad.

- Chef's salad with turkey slices, grated cheeses, olives, artichoke hearts and creamy dressing.

Dinner

- Free-range or organic charbroiled steak with steamed broccoli florets and melted butter.

- Vegan grilled tofu "pups" (low-carbohydrate variety) with mustard and mayonnaise and homemade, stevia-sweetened coleslaw.

- Grilled chicken breast with stir-fried zucchini and yellow summer squash.

- Poached salmon with fresh dill and lemon slices, served with a large artichoke, dipped in garlic mayonnaise or butter.

- Broiled lamb chops garnished with mint leaves and served with steamed cauliflower.

Snacks and Appetizers

- Raw vegetable slices with sour cream and dill dip.

- Shrimp cocktail with mayonnaise-dipping sauce (cocktail sauce contains carbohydrate).

- Half an avocado stuffed with shrimp, seasoned with garlic, lemon juice and paprika.

- Deviled eggs.
- Small handful of almonds, walnuts or macadamia nuts.

Dessert or Bedtime Snack

- Stevia-sweetened gelatin-based pudding made with whey or soy protein, stevia, cream, coconut milk and gelatin. Garnish with a dollop of (real) whipped cream.
- Halfcup strawberry slices with a dollop of whipped cream.
- Cheese plate.
- Half cup cottage cheese with fourth of a cup blueberries and stevia.
- Chocolate smoothie, made with whey protein concentrate and cocoa powder (organic, unsweetened).

• •

Hot Tip: For recipes and creative meal ideas, check out *The Smart Guide to Low-Carb Cooking* by Mia Simms and John Morgenthaler, published by Smart Publications.

• •

Keeping Track

When beginning the LCAA Diet, it is helpful to weigh and measure food and keep track of carbohydrate intake. Remember, in order to maintain ketosis, daily carbohydrate intake is best maintained within the 30-gram range (this can vary, based on individual metabolism). It is also essential to space meals, snacks and carbohydrate grams fairly evenly throughout the day. **The Bottom Line — Keep Carbohydrates Low Enough to Maintain Ketosis.**

• •

Hot Tip: Low thyroid levels can slow progress. Most people over 30 years old can benefit from a small amount of supplemental thyroid (about half a grain) even when the blood test is within the so called normal range. Check with your physician about natural thyroid supplements such as Armour, West or Biotech. Synthetic thyroid supplements such as Synthroid® can have side effects, including unwanted fluid retention.

Website: Please check our website at www.smart-publications.com. You will find information on how to order pharmaceutical products by mail from overseas (for better selection and to save money), pointers on finding a suitable physician, a subscription button for our free e-newsletter and other resources.

• •

LCAA Shopping List

We've compiled the following shopping list so you can restock your refrigerator and kitchen cupboards with low-carb foods. Have fun with this, and be sure to focus on foods you like to eat and cook with!

Vegetables and Fruits

All Leafy Green Vegetables: Arugula, baby lettuce mix, beet greens, bok choy, chard, collard greens, endive, escarole, green cabbage, green leaf lettuce, kale, Napa cabbage, red leaf lettuce, romaine lettuce, spinach.

All Non-Starchy Vegetables: Alfalfa sprouts, artichokes, asparagus, avocado, broccoli, brussels sprouts, cauliflower, celery, cucumber, eggplant, green beans, jicama, kohlrabi, leeks, mung bean sprouts, mushrooms, okra, purple cabbage, radish, rhubarb, scallions, snow pea pods, summer squash, turnips, zucchini squash. (A touch of onion adds some carbohydrate but lots of flavor, small amounts are OK.)

Canned or Condiment Vegetables: Artichoke hearts (in oil or water), bamboo shoots, hearts of palm, olives (all varieties), pickles (unsweetened only), salsa, sauerkraut, water chestnuts.

All Fresh or Dried Salad Herbs: Basil, chicory, chives, cilantro, dill, fennel, garlic, mint, onion, oregano, parsley, sage, rosemary, thyme, watercress.

Low-Carb, Low Glycemic Fruits: Strawberries, blueberries, raspberries

Meats

Coleman, Organic Valley, or other organic or free-range beef, lamb, pork, rabbit, veal, venison and other wild game. **Exceptions:** no processed meats containing sugars and/or nitrates, or other carbohydrates.

Fish: All fish, especially coldwater fish (rich in omega-3 fatty acids — see Chapter 7). Exceptions: processed fish or fish with nitrites or nitrates. Avoid imitation crab, lobster or other imitation fish.

Fowl: all organic or free-range varieties, including chicken, Cornish game hen, turkey and goose.

Exceptions: no processed poultry or products containing nitrites, nitrates, sugars or other carbohydrates.

Dairy: Organic or free-range eggs, cream, kefir (0-1 gm carbohydrate per serving), sour cream, cheeses (carbohydrate content should be 1 gm or less per ounce), whey protein concentrate

Vegan Protein Sources: Tofu, tofu flour, soy flour, low-carb soy powder, tofu cheese, rice protein powder, rice or soy cheese (check carbohydrate content), tofu sausages, texturized vegetable protein (TVP), Smart Dogs or other low-carb soy "hot dogs." Most of these products have a very low-carbohydrate content. Always check labels before buying.

Condiments: Horseradish, mayonnaise, mustard, Tabasco Sauce, Worcesshire sauce. (As with onion above, a touch of vinegar adds some carbohydrate but lots of flavor; small amounts are OK.)

Smoothie Mixes: Whey protein concentrate, soy protein powder, rice protein powder or other low-carb protein powders.

Most Nuts and Seeds: almonds, Brazil nuts, flax seeds, macadamia nuts, pecans, sunflower seeds, walnuts.

Important note: Some nuts, such as cashews, peanuts and

hazelnuts, are higher in carbohydrates. Avoid these or use them lightly as seasonings.

Oils and Fats: Whole avocado, coconut milk, flax oil*, hemp oil*, pumpkin seed oil*, olive oil*, allnut*, seed* and vegetable* oils, coconut oil, butter.

Best Oils and Fats for Cooking: Coconut oil and butter. These are naturally solid at room temperature, are able to withstand heat and are therefore best to cook and bake with. In addition, coconut oil has some surprising health benefits (see Chapter 7).

Beverages

Herb tea, green tea, decaf coffee, cream, broth or bouillon, lemon or lime juice as flavoring (1.4 gm carbohydrate per tablespoon), seltzer water, mineral water, club soda, naturally flavored water.

Sweeteners: Non-caloric herbal sweeteners, including white stevia extract, green stevia herbal powder and liquid stevia extract.**Use These Sugars and Synthetic Sweeteners With Moderation**

Sugars include all refined sugars and syrups (check for ingredients ending with -ose): glucose (dextrose), fructose, lactose (in milk), levulose, maltose (in beer) and sucrose (table sugar). Syrups made from sugar cane, sugar beets, rice, barley, sorghum, honey and maple. Synthetic sweeteners: aculfame K, saccharin and aspartame (Nutrasweet) should be avoided, since evidence suggests they may be harmful.

● ●

Hot Tip: White stevia extract is an excellent alternative to synthetic sweeteners. It is available in most health and natural food stores, and by mail order (see Resources).

Website: Please check our website at www.smart-publications.com for information on how to order nutritional products by mail (for better selection and to save

---

* Do not heat these, as it destroys their nutritional value (see Chapter 7).

money), pointers on finding a suitable physician and a subscription button for our free e-newsletter.

● ●

Chapter 5
The Skinny on Ketosis

"I s ketosis safe?" This question is common among newcomers to low-carb dieting. This chapter will put you at ease about the subject, as we present you with clinical studies that discuss the value, safety and importance of ketosis and low-carbohydrate eating. You will learn why today more than ever, physicians, clinicians and nutritionists are prescribing this type of diet for a variety of conditions.[71]

Benign Dietary Ketosis (BDK) ... is a natural, healthy response that occurs when the body switches to fat as its primary fuel source

The question of safety is often related to the confusion between deliberate dietary ketosis and *ketoacidosis,* experienced by the late-stage diabetic. Ketoacidosis in the late-stage diabetic is similar to ketosis, but it is happening for a very different reason: not because of carbohydrate restriction but because of a serious disease condition.[72] Ketosis achieved through low-carbohydrate dieting controls insulin and blood sugar levels.

Robert C. Atkins, M.D., who describes this difference in his *Dr. Atkins' New Diet Revolution,* wisely coined the term *Benign Dietary Ketosis* (BDK) to denote the beneficial state of ketosis produced through intentional low-carbohydrate eating.[73] Thus, BDK is a natural, healthy response that occurs when the body switches to fat as its primary fuel source. Clinical studies indicate that it is perfectly safe, effective and has the power to restore health, stimulate fat loss and slow down the biological clock.

Therapeutic Applications of Ketogenic Diets

Obesity, Epilepsy and Cancer

Hospitals and clinics around the world are beginning to use a ketogenic diet as a therapeutic approach for a variety of health conditions. For example, it is implemented for the dietary management of obesity for both children and adults. The diet is also prescribed to improve seizure control in children with epilepsy, especially in those who do not respond to standard medical treatment.[74] In cancer patients, the ketosis diet has been found useful in reducing tumor size and growth while maintaining the patient's nutritional status. [75]

The surprising ability of ketosis to inhibit cancer development was first detected by a group of Australian researchers, who noticed that the presence of ketone bodies inhibited malignant cell growth, and that the effects were both reversible and nontoxic. The scientists also found that dietary ketosis reduced melanoma deposits in the lungs of mice by two-thirds! These results were considered so significant that the ketogenic diet is now sometimes used as an adjunct therapy in the clinical management cancer.[76,77]

The Safety of Ketosis

To determine the overall safety of ketosis, a group of researchers placed nine lean men on a normal diet for one week, followed by a ketogenic diet for four weeks. The men consumed fewer than 20 grams of carbohydrates per day and ate a high calorie diet of protein and fat (this was not a weight loss program). The diet was well tolerated by all of the participants. Their liver and kidney functions remained healthy, and their potassium, triglyceride and cholesterol levels were virtually unchanged. Finally, the men not only maintained good health during the course of the trial, but theyalso experienced excellent reductions and balance of their blood sugar levels.[78]

Ketosis Cracks the Obesity Code

You've heard us say that the Low-Carb Anti-Aging (ketosis) Diet is the quickest, safest way to weight loss. This is especially critical for people who have suffered with obesity from an early age. In an effort to halt what usually becomes a lifelong problem, researchers placed a group of morbidly obese teen-agers, ages 12 to 15 years, on a ketosis diet. The results of the study were remarkable. Before the diet, the teens weighed an average of about 350 pounds each. After eight weeks on the very low carbohydrate diet they lost an average of 34 pounds. This was followed by 12 more weeks of a slightly higher carbohydrate program, during which they lost an additional average of five pounds.[79]

Not only did the teens lose substantial body fat (initially, an average of over four pounds a week), but their blood chemistries remained healthy and normal throughout the study. In addition, their serum cholesterol decreased from 162 to 121 during the first four weeks of the diet. And for those who had previously experienced sleep difficulties (often associated with obesity), normal sleep patterns were restored.[80]

A ketosis diet is the only one that addresses what's at the heart of many cases of obesity: hyperinsulinism (too much insulin). With the LCAA Diet or other ketosis diet, obese people actually stand a chance of leading a lean, healthy, normal life.

Low-Carb Diet More Favorable Over the Long Term

While researchers have not conducted longevity studies of low carbohydrate diets, studies do confirm their long-term safety and benefit. In one trial, 68 patients were divided into a low carbohydrate (25 percent) and a higher carbohydrate (45 percent) group. After 12 weeks, weight loss was about the same in both groups, yet the researchers concluded *"the low carbohydrate diet could be more favorable in the long term*" because of the tremendous improvements in blood chemistries, including decreases in glucose, insulin and triglycerides levels.[81]

Important Note: The LCAA Diet, which is lower in carbohydrates, would have produced a more substantial weight loss.

Another study, conducted by Elizabeth Evans, Anne Stock and John Yudkin, demonstrated all positive changes during a low-carbohydrate trial. The female participants were instructed to consume 60 grams of carbohydrates per day, with the remaining dietary intake of unlimited amounts of protein and fat. Over a period of six weeks, the women lost between 6 and 11 pounds of body fat, with no lean tissue losses. Their triglyceride, cholesterol and uric acid levels remained the same, and a small degree of ketosis was achieved. The researchers optimistically report that "the low carbohydrate diet is now widely used by physicians in many parts of the world."[82]

Better Than Fasting

Believe it or not, the LCAA Diet can produce better, faster fat loss than a total fast (no food at all). Although being in ketosis *is* a fast from carbohydrates, it is in no way a fast from eating food. Similar to a total fast, however, the body burns off its glycogen stores within the first 48 hours. By the third day of both fasting and the ketosis diet, the body's glycogen stores are burned off and the body suppresses both hunger and appetite. The major difference is that with a total fast, the body consumes its own lean tissues for fuel, while in case of ketosis, the body consumes its own fat.

One study performed at the Oakland Naval Hospital clearly demonstrated the difference between a total fast and a ketosis diet. A group of naval personnel, unable to attain their weight standards, was placed on total fast, followed by a very low carbohydrate (10 grams), high fat diet for 10 days each. During the 10-day total fast, the men lost an average of 21 pounds, which consisted of mainly lean body tissue (65 percent.) On the ketosis diet, they lost 14.5 pounds, but it was mainly body fat (97 percent), with nearly no loss of lean body mass (3 percent.) [83]

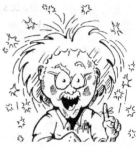

the low carbohydrate diet is now widely used by physicians in many parts of the world

Another study that compared low carbohydrate intake with fasting in 129 patients demonstrated that a ketosis diet produces rapid weight loss, the preservation of lean body tissue and no hunger. The patients lost fat at a rate of up to a half pound a day, experienced no negative effects to their blood chemistry or organ systems — including in those who continued for up to 300 days! [84]

Relief from Hypoglycemia

Hypoglycemia, the drop in blood sugar usually caused by high insulin levels, can be miserable for those who endure it. After just a few hours without food, most hypoglycemics suffer a combination of headaches, anxiety, shaking and mood fluctuations. Yet hypoglycemics who follow the LCAA Diet usually notice a complete clearance of their symptoms. Animal studies demonstrate that ketogenic diets actually have an anti-hypoglycemia effect that works by shielding the body from excessive levels of insulin. [85]

Protein for a Mental Edge

After a few days on the LCAA Diet you may find yourself in an enhanced state of mental functioning and clarity. This is mainly linked with both reduced carbohydrate intake and increased protein consumption. Clinical trials have demonstrated that carbohydrate consumption considerably decreases mental sharpness and increases drowsiness, while high-protein meals have the opposite effect. In fact, high-protein intake has consistently been shown to improve mental alertness and performance, while carbohydrates impair both performance and concentration.[86,87]

Negative Aspects of Dietary Ketosis and Solutions to Them

With all of the positive aspects of ketosis and the LCAA Diet, you might be asking yourself whether there are any negative effects to watch for. Indeed, there are some. However, they are minor when compared with the many advantages — and each one can be easily remedied. They are:

Cravings

The initial 48 hours of the diet can be very challenging as the body burns up its glycogen stores. First-timers usually experience an addictive desire for carb foods that lasts about two days. This can be helped by increasing the consumption of healthy fats (see Chapter 7). Fats not only impart a sense of satiation, but they can also induce dietary ketosis (*in the absence of carbohydrates*). In addition, an amino acid know as *L-glutamine* may be taken to relieve strong carbohydrate cravings.

• •

Safety and Precautions: L-glutamine is a natural amino acid with no known side effects.

Dosage and Timing: L-glutamine works best when taken in doses of 1,000 mg in between meals or whenever cravings occur.

Availability: L-glutamine is available in powder, capsule and tablet form. It can be purchased by mail-order and in most health and natural product stores.

• •

Halitosis

Some people experience halitosis (bad breath) as the body adjusts to the ketogenic diet. This is usually short-term and happens as ketones are released through the breath. While only few experience this, it helps to be aware that it may occur, especially during the first week on the diet. A natural antidote is parsley oil, which is an excellent breath freshener that works from the inside out.

● ●

 Safety and Precautions: Parsley oil is a plant-food derivative with no known side effects.

 Dosage and Timing: Parsley oil capsules work best when taken just after meals and may also be taken as needed. Since the individual capsule dosage will vary based on product brand, follow label instructions.

Availability: Parsley oil capsules are available at most supermarkets, drugstores and health food stores (Breath Assure® is a popular brand carried by most of these stores). Other brands are also available by mail order and in most health and natural product stores.

● ●

Constipation

For those who do not consume sufficient fiber, constipation may result. This can be relieved by increasing the amount of fiber in your diet via high fiber, low-carb vegetables (see Shopping List, Chapter 4). In addition, we recommend the use of an unsweetened fiber supplement such as psyllium husk powder and make sure you drink plenty of filtered water.

● ●

 Safety and Precautions: Psyllium husk powder is a plant-derived fiber supplement that can produce bloating and discomfort in some people. Begin with a small amount and increase dosage gradually.

Check supplement product labels to ensure it is carbohydrate-free or very low carbohydrate (some fiber supplements) with no sugar added.

Dosage and Timing: Psyllium husk powder works best when taken on an empty stomach, first thing in the morning and/or between meals. Begin with a small amount (one teaspoon) and slowly work up to one or two tablespoons daily, depending on the desired effect.

Availability: Psyllium husk products are available in most supermarkets, drugstores, and health food stores. They can also be purchased by mail-order and in most health and natural product stores.

Chapter 6
Low-Carb Superfoods

W hen most of us begin a diet — any diet — we tend to focus on what we can't have. Low-fat dieters usually miss foods such as steak, butter, eggs and cheese, while many low-carb dieters miss the breads, rice, cakes and cookies. We've found that *focusing on what you* ***can*** *have* is essential to having staying power with any diet. Many people find it easy to focus on the low-carb diet since they can eat all they want of steak, butter, eggs, cheese, cream and other fatty foods. Maybe you will be one of these people. One thing is certain, the low-carb diet is extraordinarily rich in flavor and satisfying to the appetite.

It will also help you to try out new foods, experience fresh flavors and dabble with exotic spices. To increase your food choices, this Chapter spotlights some exceptional superfoods that will titillate your taste buds as you bolster your health.

Superfood No. 1—Soy

Soy beans are a protein-rich legume that were first introduced to the United States by Benjamin Franklin. Since that time, soy foods have not been an American favorite; in fact, most soy bean crops were either imported or used as animal feed. Breaking news of soy's major health benefits, however, has sparked a nationwide soy revolution. Here's why:

The Soy Revolution

Cross-cultural and scientific studies have revealed that the humble soybean has numerous anti-aging and anti-disease attributes. The regular consumption of soy foods may reduce the risk of heart disease, lower cholesterol levels, reduce symptoms of syndrome X, decrease menopausal symptoms, prevent osteoporosis and even reduce the risk of certain types of cancer![88,89]

The Secret Is in the Isoflavones

Soy, which is commonly consumed in the Asian diet, is naturally rich in a group of compounds called *isoflavones*. These estrogen-like molecules selectively bind to certain estrogen receptors, which can produce many positive effects in both men and women. The three main isoflavones in soy are *genistein*, *daidzein* and *glycitein*. Each has its own unique group of benefits, and together they may even combat syndrome X.[90,91]

Men and women alike can benefit from the anti-estrogenic effects of soy

Soy Reverses Syndrome X

As you may recall from Chapter 1, insulin resistance is at the heart of syndrome X (the heart-disease risk factors related to high insulin levels). Remarkably, isoflavones in soy can decrease insulin levels, which, in turn, improve other facets of the syndrome, including blood lipid profiles and atherosclerosis. [92,93]

One study published in the *Lancet* further confirms soy's positive influence over syndrome X-related heart disease risks. During the study, a group of researchers replaced animal protein with soy protein in the diets of patients with high serum cholesterol. According to the results, soy significantly reduces total cholesterol, low-density lipoproteins (LDL or "bad") cholesterol and triglycerides, while minimally influencing high density lipoproteins (HDL or "good") cholesterol.[94]

More Cardiovascular Benefits

Part of what sparked the U.S. soy revolution was the epidemiological observation that Asian populations, which consume considerable amounts of soy, have a statistically lower rate of heart disease deaths than those that consume more animal protein and little or no soy protein. According to the researchers, postmenopausal women, who are at an increased risk of heart disease due to lower estrogen levels, could especially benefit from including more soy in their diets.[95]

One clinical study tested the effects of soy protein on hypertension, a major cardiovascular risk for menopausal women. The participants included 21 perimenopausal and menopausal women, each of whom received 80 milligrams of isoflavones every day for five to 10 weeks. During the study, the women's blood pressure improved so dramatically that the results were comparable to what is normally only possible with hormone replacement therapy (HRT)![96]

The Anti-Estrogen Paradox ♀

Soy isoflavones can also have a wonderfully balancing effect on the reproductive systems of women of all ages. Health professionals often recommend soy isoflavone nutritional supplements for female problems associated with estrogen imbalances, such as premenstrual syndrome (PMS), endometriosis, breast cancer and menopause symptoms — all of which stand to improve from soy isoflavone consumption.

Much of soy's positive influence on female hormones has to do with its estrogen-like activity, since isoflavones bind with certain estrogen receptors. Yet paradoxically they also are considered to have an anti-estrogenic effect which is beneficial. That's because isoflavones can reduce the body's total estrogen load by competing against more potent, problem-causing estrogens. Interestingly, postmenopausal Japanese women who eat soy foods barely suffer menopausal symptoms and are much less likely to use estrogen replacements when compared with American women who don't eat soy foods.

Anti-Cancer Potential ♂ ♀

Men and women alike can benefit from the anti-estrogenic effects of soy, since the risk of estrogen-dependent cancers is related to higher estrogen levels in both sexes. A large body of research suggests that regular soy food consumption can reduce the risk of cancers of the breast, prostate and colon.[97] In China, where soy consumption is comparatively high, women have a much lower risk of breast cancer, compared with women in Britain, where soy intake is low.[98] Other studies show that Asian men who drink alcohol, smoke cigarettes *and* consume soy foods still have lower rates of some cancers than Western men, including prostate cancer.[99]

Soy Builds Better Bones ♀

Regular soy intake even results in stronger bones! Studies of elderly Asian women who consume soy foods over a lifetime suggest that isoflavones may protect against bone loss, improve bone integrity and reduce of the risk of osteoporosis and hip fractures. In contrast, most American women experience rapid bone loss for up to 10 years following menopause. While some women resort to [synthetic] hormone replacement therapy (HRT), the side effects are often not worth the risk.* For this reason, researchers are looking to soy for safer alternatives.[100]

• •

Web site: Please check our web site at www.smart-publications.com. You will find information on how to order *Natural Hormone Replacement for Women over 45*, pointers on finding a suitable physician and a subscription button for our free e-newsletter.

• •

---

*   **Note:** Refer to *Natural Hormone Replacement* by Jonathan Wright, published by Smart Publications.

Soy Foods:

- **Balance Sex Hormones**
- **Reduce Cancer Risk**
- **Lower Total and LDL ("Bad") Cholesterol**
- **Reduce Risk of Heart Disease**
- **Prevent Osteoporosis**
- **Build Stronger Bones**

Initial clinical trials of soy's positive influence on bone density are truly promising. One double-blind, placebo-controlled, cross-over study showed that the daily consumption of just 45 milligrams of soy isoflavones increased the bone density of postmenopausal women in just 24 weeks.[101]

Soy isoflavones work to improve bone mass by activating bone cells called *osteoblasts*, which stimulate the formation of new bone tissue. In addition, soy's estrogenic effects may further contribute to the absorption and retention of bone calcium.[102]

The Bottom Line—Eat More Soy!

When consumed regularly, soy protein offers too many health benefits to pass up. Ten years ago, studies of soy protein and its isoflavones were few and far between. Today they are booming. In fact, soy has become so "hot" that the U.S. Food and Drug Administration (FDA) is even considering allowing manufacturers of soy products to use labels claiming their products may protect against heart disease.

Measurable benefits can be obtained by eating just 25 grams of soy protein a day — the equivalent of about a half cup of tofu — which, by the way, contains less than one gram of carbohydrate! With so many good tasting, low-carb soy products on the market, you'll want to be sure to eat some soy foods every day.

Safety and Precautions: In 1999, up to 65 percent of U.S. soybean crops were grown from genetically modified organism (GMO) seeds. Europeans nickname these artificial foods "Frankenstein food," and members of the European Union vehemently oppose them and have firmly banned their import. Genetically modified soybeans remain a dietary wild card. So when choosing soy products, don't gamble with a precarious unknown. Instead, look for products made from non-GMO.

Superfood No. 2 — Whey Protein Concentrate

The amino acids that make up proteins are the basic building blocks of life — and protein powders can be a great ally on the low-carb amino acid-rich diet. They are convenient for people on-the-go, can be used to make creamy, delicious low-carb "shakes" or be substituted for flour in some recipes. Protein powders are made from a variety of food sources, including whole egg, egg white, casein (from milk), soy, tofu, rice and whey (also from milk). Some are even made from beef!

While these are all good low-carb protein sources, it's important to realize that there are major differences among proteins. One in particular can significantly improve your health. It's called *whey protein concentrate* (WPC) and is the subject of nearly 15 years of research and dozens of international studies. WPC has been shown to enhance lean muscle mass, decrease body fat, stimulate immune function, prevent cancer, reduce total cholesterol and improve bone health. It can also play a key role in cell renewal and new tissue growth.

Until recently, whey protein was considered a useless byproduct of the cheese-manufacturing industry. In some cases, it was even considered unsuitable for human or animal consumption. At best, spray-dried whey powder was used as animal feed and as a bulking agent in yogurt and ice cream products. That's because most whey products contain high levels of unwanted lactose (milk sugar), fat and very little protein.

Thanks to new technological developments, today's WPC products are a gold mine of health-enhancing protein, which contain virtually no fat or lactose. Using highly specialized processing techniques, quality WPCs can contain over 90 percent of superior quality protein that is well tolerated by those who are dairy or lactose-intolerant.

Highest Biological Value

You can determine the quality of a protein based on its *biological value* (BV): The higher its BV, the more readily the body can digest, utilize and absorb it.[103] Although just about anyone can benefit from high BV proteins, they are especially important for dieters, athletes and those with compromised digestive systems such as the very old or ill (cancer, AIDs).

Surprisingly, quality whey protein concentrates have the very highest biological value on the planet (see table 6-1)! They also contain all of the essential and nonessential amino acids, with more

Table 6-1

Biologic Value (BV) of Dietary Proteins[105]

Protein Source	BV
Lactalbumin (WPC)	104
Egg	100
Cow's milk	91
Beef	80
Fish	79
Soy	74
Rice	59
Beans	49

branched chain amino acids than any other food. For dieters and athletes this translates into better, faster results. For those who are aging or diseased it can mean a second chance at life, since high BV whey protein can prevent and reverse catabolic tissue wasting.[104]

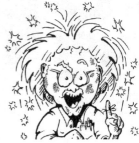

Whey protein concentrate (WPC) is the subject of nearly 15 years of research and dozens of international studies

Reduce Body Fat, Increase Lean Muscle

In a preliminary study conducted at the University of Nebraska, WPC* was shown to significantly improve body composition and strength. The 40 athletic participants were randomly divided into two groups. Group 1 received whey protein concentrate and Group 2, the control group, received a carbohydrate placebo. All 40 athletes followed the same weight-training program for four days a week. After just four weeks, the WPC group was significantly stronger and leaner than the placebo group and had lost more than double the amount of body fat. [106]

Dramatically Enhance Immune Function

When compared with other proteins, whey protein can do wonders for the immune system. WPC directly affects immunity through active components called *subfractions*. One of its most effective subfractions is *isolactoferrin*, which has powerful anti-oxidant, anti-microbial and anti-viral properties. Its other subfractions

---

*   WPC in this study was Designer Protein ™ by Next Nutrition (see Resources)

include *beta-lactoglobulin*, *alpha-lactalbumin* and*immunoglobu-lins* (IgGs).[107] Whey's most impressive immune potential, however, lies in its ability to increase *glutathione* synthesis in the body.

Glutathione—
Antioxidant at Large

Next to vitamin C, glutathione has been called the most influential antioxidant in the entire body. This compound protects the cells against free radicals and neutralizes toxins, such as heavy metals, carcinogens and peroxides. It is also involved in numerous physio-logical processes, including healthy immune function, DNA and protein synthesis, enzyme activity and drug metabolism.[108]

WPC raised glutathione levels more effectively and consistently than any other protein

While glutathione is essential to good health, it is not efficient as an oral supplement because the body breaks much of it down before it can be utilized. Glutathione is made from glutamate, cysteine and glycine, three amino acids which are con-nected together to form glutathione. Since digestion breaks down proteins, even small peptides like glutathione, oral intake of glutathione is inefficient. Fortunately, the body is fairly efficient at making its own glutathione, and whey protein concentrate may be the best way to help it do so. In animal studies, WPC raised glu-tathione levels more effectively and consistently than any other pro-tein.[109] This is because WPC contains glutamylcysteine, which is two-thirds of the glutathione molecule. Glutamylcysteine is readily converted into glutathione by the body.

Cancer Protection

Additional research suggests that dietary whey protein may also protect against cancer and various tumors in humans and animals.[110,111] A recent study also showed that WPC helped boost the recovery of cancer patients. The researchers reported: "Whey's anti-oxidant and tumor preventive abilities...[can] work synergistically with other forms of anti-cancer therapy, stimulate the host's immune system, and potentially scavenge remaining microscopic cancer cells."[112]

 whey protein can do wonders for the immune system.

WPC Lowers Cholesterol

Other research shows that whey protein concentrate is remarkably effective at lowering cholesterol levels — even better than soy! In a study comparing WPC, casein and soybeans, WPC was found to lower cholesterol 20 percent better than casein and 38 percent more effectively than soybeans.[113] Another study showed that WPC reduced elevated blood pressure 10 percent more effectively than soy.[114]

Bone Health Benefits

Whey protein can even play a role in improving bone density. As with soy, WPC seems to activate the bone-forming cells called *osteoblasts*. Researchers have also found that it positively affects collagen, the main connective tissue in bones (and in body).[115] Studies have yet to prove whether whey protein can prevent or reverse the cross-linking of collagen (see Chapter 2).

Whey Protein Concentrate

- Boosts immune function
- Builds lean body tissue
- Enhances collagen formation
- Increases glutathione levels
- Inhibits cancer and tumor growth
- Promotes fat loss
- Protects against free radical damage
- Strengthens bones

Look for Advanced WPC Formulas

The best whey protein concentrates utilize low-temperature processing methods that produce an isolate that is over 90 percent protein and virtually 100 percent undenatured (undamaged). This means that its subfractions remain concentrated and biologically active, which is essential to its many benefits (see Resources).

Superfood No. 3—Vegetables!

Fresh, organically grown vegetables are low in carbohydrates, calories and fat, yet rich in health-promoting vitamins, minerals, antioxidants, enzymes, flavonoids, fiber and phytochemicals. In addition to their potent anti-aging benefits, these natural foods can lower the risk of many diseases. For example, the addition of just one vegetable serving a day can reduce the risk of colorectal cancer by more than 20 percent.[116] Vegetable-rich diets also reduce the risk of coronary heart disease, osteoporosis and age-related vision loss.[117] Mother was really right when she insisted that you "Eat your vegetables!"

Phytochemical Power

Beyond the basic nutrients found in vegetables, these foods contain an abundance of compounds known as *phytochemicals*. These are powerful substances found in all plant life (*phyto* means plant), some of which have been identified as *dithiolthiones, glucosinolates, indoles, isothiocyanates, flavonoids, phenols, protease inhibitors, plant sterols, allium compounds, limonen.* While researchers have identified some of these disease-fighting substances, many remain unidentified.[118]

broccoli, cauliflower, cabbage and Brussels sprouts, are among the most potent of the anti-cancer vegetables

Phytochemicals are the unique non-nutritive components in plants that appear to have special medicinal effects in the body. Some lower cholesterol, inhibit blood clotting or control allergies, while others can reduce inflammation, restrict tumor growth, and even regenerate organ systems. Phytochemicals also have powerful anticarcinogenic (anti-cancer) properties.[119]

Anti-Cancer Cruciferous Vegetables

The cruciferous vegetable group, including broccoli, cauliflower, cabbage and Brussels sprouts, are among the most potent of the anti-cancer vegetables. These low-carb veggies stand apart for their naturally rich phytochemical content.

Currently, researchers are especially focused on a specific cruciferous phytochemical, known as *indole-3-carbinol* (I3C). This compound, which positively influences estrogen metabolism in humans, could make a major impact on the war against cancer. Recent findings show that I3C can inhibit breast cancer cell growth by 90 percent — 30 percent better than the newly FDA-approved drug, tamoxifen, which inhibits breast cancer cell growth by 60 percent.[120,121] This is very exciting news.

Cruciferous vegetables have many other benefits, including a beneficial influence on cardiovascular health. One recently published study evaluated the fruit and vegetable intake of over 34,000 postmenopausal women. When the results were tallied, only broccoli was strongly associated with a marked reduction of coronary heart disease risk.[122]

The Powers of Green

When it comes to maximum nutrition for minimal carbohydrate content, the leafy green vegetables are the best deal around. These power-packed veggies include spinach, chard, kale, arugula and a variety of lettuces and herbs. They are virtually devoid of calories and fat, yet chock-full of vitamins, minerals (potassium, magnesium, calcium and many trace minerals), enzymes, fiber, chlorophyll, and carotenes. Also rich in antioxidants and other cancer-protective agents, these versatile vegetables are remarkably healthy foods.[123] We suggest eating them daily.

Boost Immunity with the Allium Family

Since the times of the earliest Chinese dynasties and of Ancient Egypt, garlic (*Allium sativum*) has served as both food and medicine. This exceptional bulb belongs to the *allium* family of vegetables, which includes onions, scallions, leeks and chives. Recognized for their traditional and medicinal benefits, these pungent vegetables have been the topic of over 2,000 research articles over the past 24 years.[124]

The sulfur-rich allium family of vegetables is best known for its potent antibacterial and immune-enhancing effects. More recent interest in allium phytochemical compounds has focused on their potential to reduce blood pressure, cholesterol levels and other cardiovascular risks.[125] They may also remove toxic heavy metals from the body, protect neurons and inhibit damage from free radicals. In addition, their anti-carcinogenic properties may reduce the risk of some cancers, including stomach and colon cancer.[126]

Beyond their impressive health benefits, these flavorful vegetables can make food taste great. Enjoy their hearty flavor by adding them to your favorite recipes. These and many other vegetables may be eaten liberally on the LCAA Diet — and should comprise the bulk of your carbohydrate intake. Also, try using fresh herbs such as basil, cilantro, rosemary and thyme. They do wonders to enhance the taste of food and also contain phytochemicals of their own.

Chapter 7
Anti-Aging Fats to Grow Lean By
Cure Your Fat Phobia!

Most Americans have been convinced that any amount and any kind of fat is unhealthy. A principle advertising strategy for carb-loaded products is to promote their fat-free status, implying that fat has health risks that non-fat foods are lower-calorie and healthier choices. However, new information is proving that many fats are not only valuable but essential to good health. In fact, many can help reverse life-threatening conditions, including syndrome-X-related heart disease, hypertension, atherosclerosis and type II diabetes.[127,128,129]

In addition, certain fats can improve your results on the LCAA Diet, induce dietary ketosis and even improve metabolism. This chapter focuses on those fats that can enhance health and extend life span and also informs you about which fats are important to avoid.

The Fat-Free Blues

Have you ever started a low- or no-fat diet and found yourself struggling with gnawing hunger and lack of energy? Many fat-free programs have this effect, which is why most people don't continue with them. Those who do continue risk damaging delicate fat-dependent tissues, including the brain and nervous system, which rely on fatty acids for their cellular make-up.[130] Over the years, fat-restricted diets can actually lead to premature aging, and fat-free folks often begin looking, feeling and functioning older than their age.

Conditions that Could Indicate EFA Deficiency

- Arthritis
- Behavioral problems
- Cardiovascular disease
- Dry skin or eczema
- High cholesterol levels
- Hormone imbalances
- Growth retardation
- Immune weakness
- Male sterility
- Menstrual problems
- Organ degeneration
- Premature death

The Friendly Aspects of Fat

Newcomers to the LCAA Diet may find it astonishing that an anti-aging diet allows for unrestricted fat intake. But fats have many important functions on this diet, and, in the absence of carbohydrates, they can do you a world of good.[131] Physiologically, fats provide the foundation of many hormones in the body and are required for the structure of each and every cell wall. They are necessary for the transport of fat-soluble nutrients, including vitamins A, E, D, K, and beta carotene. As mentioned earlier, they are essential for the brain and nerve tissues as well.

Avoid the Randle Effect

Fats only present a problem to the dieter when they are consumed with carbohydrates. The Randle effect, or the competition between carbohydrate and fat utilization, causes the body to burn the fat for fuel while rapidly converting carbohydrates into glucose, triglycerides, cholesterol and stored fat.[132] However, when carbs are left out of the equation, fats provide fuel, suppress the appetite and help maintain cellular health.[133]

EFAs for Health and Weight Loss

Some fats are vital to anti-aging. Known as essential fatty acids (EFAs), they include two polyunsaturated fats: *linoleic* (an omega-6 oil) and *alpha-linolenic acid* (an omega-3 oil). They are termed as "essential" because the body cannot make them, yet they are critical to every cell of the body. Here's how:

EFAs are also the building blocks of an entire class of hormones called prostaglandins. These prostaglandins coordinate many aspects of tissue-level defense to injuries involving oxidative stress (wounds, bruises, burns, abrasion).

Our very first EFAs come from mother's milk which is a source of EPA and DHA, which are laid down in brain membranes. These fats are not found in cow's milk. Thereafter, they must be derived from foods. Some good sources include fish oil, some vegetable oils, seeds and nuts. The regular consumption of EFAs can aid weight loss, enhance mental functioning, improve energy production and promote overall health; yet an estimated 80 percent of our population does not get enough.[134]

Fish Oils for Omega 3s

Hundreds of studies have demonstrated the importance of omega-3-rich fish oils in the diet. They have had favorable effects on insulin resistance, cardiovascular health, glucose intolerance, type II diabetes, autoimmune diseases, and chronic inflammatory diseases.[135,136,137] Numerous population studies correlate an omega-3-rich diet with a significantly lower risk of heart disease, and the oils can also help to prevent the onset of a heart attack.[138,139] One recent study evaluated this heart connection in over 76,000 postmenopausal women and found that those who consumed diets rich in omega-3 fatty acids had the lowest incidence of fatal heart attacks.[140]

According to Julian Whitaker, M.D., best-selling author of *Shed 10 Years in 10 Weeks,* fish oil can help prevent heart attack and stroke by discouraging the formation of blood clots. He claims that the regular consumption of fish oil can also reduce blood pressure, cholesterol and triglyceride levels, and states, "I have observed triglyceride levels in my patients fall from over 1,000 to less than 200, simply by supplementing with fish oil."[141]

Eat More Fish!

If you like the taste of fish, you may want to consider eating more of it — especially in light of some recent findings. One comparison study found that increasing fish consumption yielded better health results than taking fish oil capsules.[142,143] This may be because fish oil is protected from rancidity while extracted fish oil may become peroxidized while inside the gelatin capsule. Another study showed that fish consumption combined with weight loss programs substantially reduces cardiovascular risk, blood pressure and heart rate in overweight hypertensives.[144]

The best fish choices for omega-3 fatty acids include the coldwater variety from unpolluted waters, such as salmon, herring, rainbow trout, sardines, eel and mackerel. If you are vegetarian or do not enjoy the taste of fish, you can increase your omega-3s by eating more flax oil or by eating freshly ground flax seed. (Omega-3 from flax, however, is a shorter-chain omega-3 fatty acid which can be changed into arachidonic acid, unlike the longer-chain EPA and DHA which cannot. So in terms of fatty acid balance in the body, fish oil is better.)

Flax Oil Has Similar Benefits

While the bulk of omega-3 research is on fish oil, you can achieve similar results by increasing your flax oil consumption. Flax seeds, from which the oil is made, are the richest natural source of omega-3 fatty acids. Studies have shown that the oil offers the same protective effects against cardiovascular disease as fish oil, and it is also effective in reducing platelet aggregation (blood clotting which can lead to heart attack or stroke).[145]

Fresh flax oil has a delicious, buttery taste and can be poured over steamed vegetables, used in salad dressings or added to low-carb blender drinks. Ounce for ounce, flax is also much more cost effective than fish oil.

• •

Safety and Precautions: Many fish oil capsules may already be oxidized (spoiled) before you even take them. Therefore, eating fresh fish is the best way to be sure that your fish oil is of high quality.

Also, much flax oil on the market may already be oxidized (rancid, spoiled) before you even buy it. If it tastes or smells bad, you know it is spoiled but this, alone, is not a reliable measure. A fairly high degree of dangerous oxidation can be present without the oil tasting or smelling bad. The only way to be certain of getting high quality oil is to eat the fresh, raw flax seed available in most health food stores. You can simply chew them up or grind them in a coffee grinder right before eating. Or you might mix them into a blender drink and let the blender grind them. (If you eat them without somehow grinding them first, they will not get digested properly.)

Hot Tip: For a delicious, health-promoting drink that tastes like a milkshake, combine soy and/or whey protein concentrate (vanilla or other flavor) with flax oil or flax seed, stevia, ice and purified water. Blend for two minutes and enjoy.

• •

Flax Oil — Handle With Care

If you do wish to use flax oil (rather than seed), freshness is imperative. This oil is easily destroyed by heat (cooking), air, light and chemicals. Look for cold-pressed flax oil pressed from organic seeds and stored in the refrigerated section of the store. Read the label to make sure the oil has been processed in the absence of heat, air and light, and packaged in dark, opaque nitrogen-sealed bottles.

• •

Hot Tip: Before purchasing flax oil, check the press date to make sure it's fresh (dated within one to two months). Once opened, keep it fresh by storing it in the refrigerator, or, better yet, in the freezer. It will not freeze solid and will last up to a year. It is also a good idea to taste it before each use. It should always taste pleasant. If it has an acrid bite to the back center of your tongue {possibly producing a mild gagging reflex}, it is rancid and should be discarded. Waste can be avoided by buying small-sized containers and using it up quickly.

• •

Surprising News About Tropical Oils

Tropical oils have received a bad rap over the years. They have become the underdog in the world of fats and are widely thought to increase triglycerides, cholesterol and other heart disease risk factors. Upon closer examination, however, we found that quite the opposite is true.

Epidemiological studies show that natural tropical oils, used in the countries of their origin, do not appear to have these negative effects. Instead they appear to boast major health benefits. *The Demographic Yearbook* of the United Nations reports that *Sri Lanka, where coconut oil is the main source of dietary fat, has the very lowest death rate due to heart disease!* [146]

Coconut Oil Activates the Metabolism

According to biochemical researcher and writer Ray Peat, Ph.D., whose primary work is focused on the endocrine system, coconut oil activates the metabolism and supports thyroid function. Peat states that "The anti-obesity effect of coconut oil is clear in all of the animal studies, and in my friends who eat it regularly...I found that eating more coconut oil lowered my weight...and eating less [coconut oil] caused it to increase."[147]

In the 1940s, farmers tried using coconut oil as a cheap method of fattening their livestock. Instead they found that the oil produced leaner, hungrier and more active animals.[148] Additional research shows that the regular consumption of coconut oil reduces "white fat" stores in animals, and that it lowers total and LDL cholesterol in people with elevated cholesterol levels.[149,150]

Sri Lanka, where coconut oil is the main source of dietary fat, has the very lowest death rate due to heart disease!

The Magic of Coconut Oil Is in the MCTS

Coconut oil contains significant amounts of a type of fat called *medium-chain triglyceride* (MCT). MCT is a highly specialized oil that reduces body fat, reverses arteriosclerosis, improves glucose metabolism and even lowers serum and liver cholesterol while raising HDLs (the "good" cholesterol). Of all the fats and oils, coconut oil is nature's richest natural source, containing over 50 percent MCT.[151]

MCTs Induce Ketosis

Numerous clinics and hospitals use MCTs to support the state of ketosis in their patients requiring this special diet. For example, the Columbia Presbyterian Medical Center Babies and Children's Hospital of New York relies on MCTs to induce ketosis. According to researchers Carroll and Koenigsberger, the majority of patients at the hospital "find our diet more acceptable and/or more user friendly than other types of ketogenic diets."[152] Other researchers report that a 60 percent MCT, 20 percent protein and 10 percent carbohydrate, and 10 percent other fat diet is the most successful in producing ketosis.*[153]

MCTs can now be purchased in a liquid, concentrated form; however, we recommend cooking with coconut oil and coconut milk, since MCT oils are highly processed and expensive. Also, coconut oil can be brought to a higher temperature before smoking so it is better for high temperature frying although MCTs are fine for low temperature cooking such as frying an egg. Coconut oil contains about 50 percent MCTs, is inexpensive, and very heat-stable — making it one of the best possible fats for cooking and frying.

Use Only Heat-Stable Fats for Cooking

When liquid vegetable oils are heated, as when cooking and baking, and especially frying and sautéeing, they undergo chemical changes that render them harmful. This is called peroxidation or rancidification. To avoid this, always use butter and/or coconut oil (available in most natural food stores) which are safe to heat, even at -high temperatures.

---

*   **Important Note:** These diets are extreme because they are used therapeutically. The moderate consumption of coconut oil and other fats will sufficiently induce ketosis on the LCAA Diet.

● ●

Hot Tip: For any oil-containing recipes requiring heat, remember this rule of thumb: If it is *naturally* solid at room temperature (butter, palm and coconut oils), it is safe to heat and eat; otherwise, do not heat it.

● ●

Cholesterol Concerns

The word "cholesterol" often draws a negative reaction because few realize that cholesterol is actually essential for health — and for life itself. More of a waxy alcohol than a fat, cholesterol is an important building block for various hormones, such as estrogen and testosterone. Along with the EFAs, it helps the body absorb fat-soluble vitamins (A, D, E, K, and beta carotene) and also allows the brain and nervous system to transmit electrical signals.

Because the body needs a certain amount of cholesterol to stay healthy, medical professionals watch for abnormally low cholesterol levels as a potential indicator of diseases such as cancer.

Insulin Triggers Cholesterol Production

If your cholesterol levels are high, you may have noticed that a reduction in dietary cholesterol does not necessarily bring them down. That's because up to 80 percent of the cholesterol in your blood is made by your own cells, primarily in the liver. One of the lesser known facts about cholesterol is that *insulin activates the cholesterol-making process*. In other words, insulin, not dietary fat, is the primary cause of elevated serum cholesterol.[154]

With your new low-carb approach to eating, however, your insulin levels will come down naturally. As a result, you should notice a gradual reduction of your serum cholesterol as well. Remember, most of your cholesterol is made by the liver and only about 20 percent comes from dietary cholesterol.

For peace of mind, have your blood cholesterol checked before and during the LCAA Diet. You should notice it drop to a healthy 180 to 200 mg/dl range, with an LDL/HDL ratio of under 3. And according to Dr. Atkins, the extra fat in your diet should also cause a rise in the HDL ("good") cholesterol.[155]

Go for Organic Meat and Dairy

When it comes to animal foods, our concern is not so much the increased fat and cholesterol as it is the high level of chemicals in most of today's meats. Most livestock is fed pesticide-, herbicide- and fungicide-laced feed, and the animals are usually injected with growth hormones and antibiotics. Traces of these chemicals in food are permitted by the FDA.

In contrast, certified organic meat, poultry, eggs and dairy products are produced without these toxic chemicals. Farmers like George Siemon of Organic Valley (a line of organic beef, eggs and dairy products — see Resources) allow their cattle to graze in open pastures and munch on organic feed. According to Siemon, "Organic farming requires that farmers develop a relationship with their livestock and the land."[156] The end result is healthier animals, healthier people and less reason to be concerned about Mad Cow Disease! If you cannot find organic livestock products locally, look for companies that will deliver them by overnight mail.

Fats to Avoid—Processed, Refined and Altered Fats

Some fats are harmful, and on the LCAA Diet it is important to know which ones they are. Unhealthy fats are those that are processed, commercially refined or chemically altered. These fats and the foods that contain them make up the bulk of fat consumption in our Western diet. They can be found in fast food, deep-fried foods, baked goods, processed convenience foods and candies.

Most supermarket oils belong in this category. Many are processed, oxidized, hydrogenated, deodorized, bleached, de-gummed or otherwise damaged. These are no longer "essential" oils.

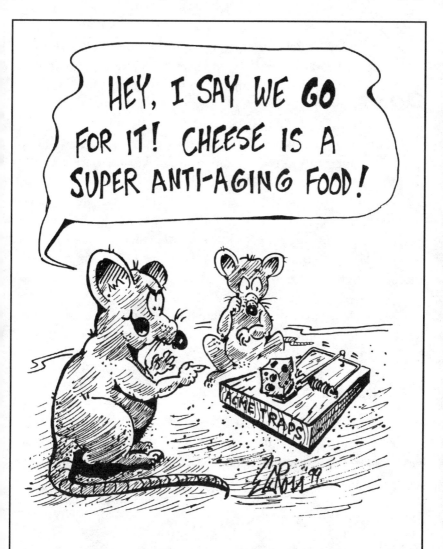

About the only case in which a low-carb diet might lead to trouble!

Parkay or Butter?

Many people grew up believing that margarine was better than butter. However, margarine contains a type of fat called *trans-fat*. The process of hydrogenation converts regular unsaturated fatty acids to trans-fatty acids, which are unnatural and play a role in major diseases such as heart disease.[157] Even "healthy" margarines and those marked "cholesterol-free" contain trans-fatty acids that should be avoided. Whenever you see "hydrogenation" or "partial hydrogenation" on a food label, there is trans fat in the product.

A recent follow-up of the well-known Framingham Study showed a strong link between margarine intake and coronary heart disease (CHD). The study tracked 832 men — who were free of coronary heart disease when the study began (it is continuing). During the 21-year follow-up, about a third (267) of the men had suffered a previous heart attack. When the men's margarine and butter intake was compared, the results showed that margarine significantly increased the risk of heart attack. Interestingly, butter did not play a role in heart attack prediction at all![158] Other studies of margarine and trans-fatty acids link their consumption to premature aging and to the development of atherosclerosis, cancers, tumors and other serious illnesses. [159] [160]

Oxidized Fats

Oxidized fats are fats that have been excessively heated or have spoiled.* They are most commonly found in processed, cured and aged foods such as sausages, luncheon meats, some cheeses, fried foods and packaged convenience foods. Your best bet is to simply avoid these foods and stick with fresh, wholesome items such as those listed on the Low-Carb Shopping List (see Chapter 4).

Focus on Healthy Fats

Be sure to look for fresh, cold-pressed oils, which can be purchased at health and natural food stores, made from organically grown nuts, seeds and coconut. Get your omega-3 fatty acids from cold

---

*   Fats become spoiled when they react with oxygen. This may be due to aging, processing, simple air exposure or storage without antioxidant protection. Antioxidants intercept oxygen-free radicals before they can attack fats and damage them.

water fish and/or flax seed or oil (hemp oil, available in health foods stores, is another good source). For cooking and baking, use butter or coconut oil. Remember that coconut oil induces (accelerates) ketosis, increases energy metabolism and, surprisingly, may protect against heart disease.

Hot Tip: All oils that are liquid at room temperature should be refrigerated to deter rancidity.

Chapter 8
Insulin-Smart Anti-Aging Supplements

If you do nothing but follow the LCAA Diet described in Chapter 4, you cannot help but reap benefits from this book. But what if we told you there was something extra you could do to speed your progress? In our research, we have uncovered some very special supplements that can restore insulin sensitivity, balance blood sugar and even reverse some of the damage caused by insulin resistance. While nutritional supplementation is an optional part of this program, you may find its anti-aging aspects too tempting to pass up.

"Anti-syndrome X" Antioxidants

With syndrome X, the body is out of balance, which creates an environment that literally generates free *radicals:* highly destructive molecules that inflict damage to healthy cells by "stealing" electrons from them. When left unchecked, free radicals play a significant role in the development of heart disease and other degenerative diseases.[161] They can, however, be controlled through the adequate intake of *antioxidant* nutrients. These include vitamins, minerals and other compounds that protect the body by donating electrons to "quench" or neutralize free radicals.

Antioxidant Deficiencies and Heart Disease

The importance of antioxidant nutrition was recently demonstrated in a large European study. The trial revealed that Finland, Central and Eastern European countries have recently experienced a tremendous increase in premature cardiovascular death rates — exceeding even those of the United States. Because free radicals are known to destroy the delicate vascular system, researchers suspect antioxidant deficiency as a significant cause and are now referring to it as a "new cardiovascular risk factor." While further studies of free antioxidant deficiencies (vitamins C, E, carotenoids and flavonoids) and cardiovascular disease are underway, we're not waiting for the results.[162] Plenty of studies have already proven the protective benefits of antioxidant nutrients, and we suggest you take them as well.

Antioxidants Combat Cross-Linking

Free radical destruction is most obvious in the type II diabetic, whose chronically high blood sugar levels is the major factor underlying glycation and the cross-linking of collagen (see Chapter 2).[163] The good news is that regular antioxidant use can reverse or inhibit some of this damage. So far, superoxide dismutase (SOD) and vitamins C and E have been identified as the most effective antioxidants against cross-linking.[164] These may be even more effective when taken with pyridoxine (vitamin B-6) and thiamine (vitamin B-1). Combined, the nutrients can provide excellent protection against the free-radical damage, the production of AGEs (advanced glycation end products) and the cross-linking of collagen.[165]

Alpha Lipoic Acid (ALA)— An Exceptional Antioxidant

With end-stage syndrome X, or type II diabetes, chronically high insulin and glucose levels are known to inflict extensive nerve damage to its victims. It is now possible to prevent or reverse some of this damage with a unique fat- and water-soluble antioxidant known as *alphalipoic acid* (lipoate). While every body produces some natural quantities of lipoate, diabetics and heart disease patients produce inadequate levels of it.[166]

In Europe, doctors administer lipoate to their patients to restore nerve health, blood sugar balance and to halt retinal degeneration.[167] In Germany, it is prescribed for the treatment of diabetic neuropathy. The regular use of this antioxidant protects the nerve tissues and may even regenerate damaged nerves.[168]

One double-blind, placebo-controlled study demonstrated just how well ALA works against diabetic neuropathy. A total of 328 type II diabetics were suffering the typical symptoms of nerve damage, including burning, numbness and discomfort in their hands or feet. After just three weeks of ALA supplementation, the patients experienced a 30 percent reduction of their total symptoms.[169] In a similar study, ALA's effects were compared against vitamin E, selenium and a placebo. Although the ALA group experienced the best results, vitamin E and selenium also resulted in substantial improvements.[170]

This potent antioxidant is not just for diabetics. It is also an excellent anti-aging supplement and is able to recycle vitamins C and E after they have been used up in free radical reactions.[171] Regular ALA supplementation may also reduce the incidence of cataracts and glaucoma, improve glucose metabolism, restore brain and liver health, prevent nerve disorders and offer protection against cigarette smoke, heavy metals and radiation damage.[172]

● ●

Safety and Precautions: In cases of severe thiamine (vitamin B-1) deficiency, high ALA intake may be toxic.[173] Lipoate works closely with thiamine in the body. It is therefore a good idea to make sure your supplement program includes some thiamine when taking this supplement. Only a few cases of skin conditions have been reported as potential side effects. Lipoate is a growth factor for bacteria, so it might also be a good idea not to take lipoate during an active infection. (This proscription also applies to iron, copper, zinc and tryptophan.)

Dosage and Timing: Therapeutic dosages of ALA range from 100-600 mg a day.

Availability: In the United States, alpha lipoic acid is considered a nutritional supplement and is available at health and natural product stores, and by mail order.

• •

Chromium and Vanadium— Two Trace Minerals That Work Well Together

Chromium and vanadium are two trace minerals which have a remarkably positive effect on insulin and blood sugar levels. Studies continue to determine that when chromium levels are low, glucose intolerance worsens, and vice versa.[174] Likewise, a growing body of research validates vanadium's potential role in improving glucose tolerance and insulin sensitivity.

Chromium Allows Insulin to be More Effective

Chromium is an essential trace mineral that is required for carbohydrate metabolism and insulin sensitivity. It is the unique component of a blood-sugar-regulating molecule called Glucose Tolerance Factor (GTF), which works intimately with insulin to facilitate the uptake of glucose into the cells, helping insulin to do a better job. Deficiencies of this important element are directly related to insulin resistance, hyperglycemia (elevated blood sugar), type II diabetes, atherosclerosis and cardiovascular disease.[175]

The profound importance of chromium for diabetics has been indicated by numerous clinical trials. One double-blind study of type I- and II- diabetics showed that just 10 days of chromium picolinate supplementation allowed 73 percent of the patients to reduce their medications. Some of the type I diabetics were even able to reduce their insulin requirements by as much as 30 percent (the placebo group showed no changes).[176]

Another study showed that chromium picolinate can also reduce blood sugar, insulin and cholesterol levels as well as levels of a compound called *glycated hemoglobin* (a longer-term measure of blood sugar). The double-blind placebo-controlled trial compared various dosages and found the 500 microgram (mcg) dosage to produce the best results.[177]

Chromium Picolinate for Fat Loss

In the natural supplements market, chromium is most popular as a weight loss agent. However, some skeptics still doubt whether it really works. While it may not work overnight, research indicates that it decreases body fat and protects against lean tissue losses. In a 90-day double-blind clinical trial, participants taking 400 micrograms of the mineral lost 17 pounds of body fat but no lean tissue. The placebo controls lost over half a pound of lean tissue and only about 3 pounds of fat.[178]

• •

 Safety and Precautions: A recent edition of the *Berkeley Wellness Letter* makes a case against chromium, stating that chromium is toxic. It is critical to point out that the researchers cited neither human nor animal studies. Instead these were test tube studies of hamster cells exposed to an equivalent of 3,000 times the recommended amount of chromium.[179] To our knowledge, there are no known side effects or toxicity of chromium when taken at the recommended dosages.

 Dosage and Timing: 400-600 mcg of chromium picolinate or chromium polynicotinate per day, taken with meals.

 Availability: Chromium is a nutritional supplement

available at health and natural product stores, and by mail order.

● ●

Vanadium Mimics Insulin!

Vanadium, named after the goddess of beauty, luster and youth, is usually acknowledged for its importance in bone and tooth formation. One of its more recently recognized functions is that *it can safely and effectively mimic insulin*. In fact, vanadium is so good at duplicating the actions of insulin, that researchers are seriously considering its role in the fight against diabetes.[180]

This may have you wondering: "If insulin is essentially a poison, why should I take a mineral that mimics it?" Because vanadium works like a back-door key that copies only the positive actions of insulin. Through alternative routes, it allows glucose and other nutrients into the cells, even when insulin has lost its ability to do so.[181]

This wonder mineral is so effective at duplicating insulin that it is often referred to as "antidiabetic, anithyperglycemic and insulinomimetic."[182] According to research at the University of British Columbia in Vancouver, sufficient doses of vanadyl sulfate (one form of the mineral) completely eliminated diabetes in laboratory animals.[183] Another animal study showed that vanadium may help preserve and protect pancreatic beta-cells.[184]

In short-term human studies, vanadium shows similar positive effects. One study of an oral form of the mineral found that it reduces both insulin resistance and fasting glucose levels in type II diabetics. [185] In another trial of type II diabetics, vanadyl sulfate improved insulin sensitivity and [muscle] glycogen by about 30 percent in just three weeks. According to the researchers, the results "were sustained for up to two weeks after the supplement was discontinued."[186]

Best Taken as Vanadyl Sulfate

Vanadium can be be found in trace amounts in a variety of foods, such as soybeans, shellfish, mushrooms and many vegetables, black pepper, dill and parsley. However, the dietary intake of most people is not usually sufficient to reproduce the therapeutic effects reflected by the research.[187] Most people can benefit by taking vanadyl sulfate orally as a daily supplement.[188]

●●●●●●●●●●●●●●●●●●●●●●●●●●●●●●●●●●●●●

Safety and Precautions: Excessive doses of vanadate (but not vanadyl sulfate) can increase blood pressure, reduce coenzyme Q10 and coenzyme A levels, stimulate MAO inhibitors and interfere with energy production. High levels have also been linked to manic depression.[189]

Diabetics who are currently taking medication for their condition should only take the mineral under a physician's supervision.

Dosage and Timing: Therapeutic dosages of vanadyl sulfate range from 50 to 150 micrograms.

Availability: Vanadyl sulfate is a nutritional supplement and is available at health and natural product stores, and by mail order.

●●●●●●●●●●●●●●●●●●●●●●●●●●●●●●●●●●●●

Gymnema Sylvestre

Gymnema sylvestre is an herb originating in East India, where it has long been used to control diabetes. Its common name, *gurmar*, means "sugar-destroying," which refers to its ability to suppress the sweet taste of sugar after the herb has been chewed. Its true effectiveness, however, lies in its potential to control blood sugar in both humans and animals. In some cases, the regular use of Gymnema has eliminated the need for hypoglycemic drugs in human diabetics.

One study of Gymnema involved 22 type II diabetics, all of whom were taking prescribed medications to control their blood sugar. They received a daily liquid extract of the herb and were monitored closely for changes. During the 20-month study, all of the patients exhibited major reductions in blood glucose levels, and five of the 22 were able to discontinue their medication and maintain their blood sugar levels using just the herbal extract.[190]

In a similar study, researchers tested the effects of a Gymnema extract on insulin-dependent (type I) diabetics. As in the previous study, daily doses of the herb caused a gradual decrease of blood glucose, and the participants' medication requirements (insulin injections) were also reduced.[191]

● ●

Safety and Precautions: Gymnema sylvestre is generally considered safe and non-toxic. Diabetics who are taking medication for their condition should take the herb only under a physician's supervision.

Dosage and Timing: Gymnema sylvestre comes in a variety of forms, including liquid extracts, tablets, capsules and teas. Since potencies may vary from product to product, it is best to follow dosage instructions on the label or to work with a knowledgeable health practitioner.

Availability: Gymnema sylvestre is an herbal nutritional supplement and is available at health and natural product stores, and by mail order.

● ●

Water—So Simple, So Necessary

Next to oxygen, water is our most essential requirement for life. With the LCAA Diet, sufficient water is especially important for several reasons. As the ketosis mobilizes fat molecules, toxins that have accumulated in the fatty tissues are also released. Drinking enough water ensures the safe and natural removal of these waste products. In addition, adequate water intake is necessary for an accurate assessment of ketosis, since concentrated urine can skew Lipostix® readings (see Chapter 4).

Water Is the Best Disease Prevention

Water is also important for longevity and disease prevention. In his book, *Your Body's Many Cries for Water*, F. Batmanghelidj, M.D., describes how chronic, unintentional dehydration is at the root of many serious afflictions, including asthma, hypertension, arthritis, high cholesterol, edema and even diabetes. Without sufficient water, the body attempts to secure its fluid supply by holding onto sodium to maintain fluid balance. This can result in excess fluid retention (edema), which is often a sign of dehydration![192]

As the body increasingly loses water and enters a dehydrated state, it is also forced gradually and systematically to close down its capillary beds. This is the only way the system can continue to support life. When water is scarce, some parts of the body, such as the brain, actually have a "priority" status, while some cells go without having their basic needs met. [193]

Anti-Aging Tonic Par Excellence

Sufficient water is not only important for disease prevention, it is genuinely the best "anti-aging" agent around. Consider that when we are born our bodies are nearly 90 percent water. As we age, this can drop to as low as 60 percent — if we don't drink enough water. Some of its most important functions include the distribution of nutrients and chemical messages throughout the body. Water also maintains body temperature, acts as a "shuttle" for important minerals and flushes metabolic toxins from the system. In fact, every cellular function is monitored by and depends upon the adequate supply of water.

Make Sure to Drink Enough

The amount of water contained by your body depends on the balance between your total water intake and excretion. The body naturally releases an average of about two quarts of water a day in the form of sweat, exhalation and urination. Factors that lead to further losses include alcohol, coffee, tea and other caffeinated beverages, as well as physical activity and heat. In addition, conditions such as diarrhea, kidney disease and diabetes also contribute to water loss.

Most people have heard and read about the importance of drinking eight to 10 eight-ounce glasses of water (64-80 ounces) per day, yet many do not even come close to consuming this amount. This may seem like a lot to drink, but it is just the right amount to keep you hydrated. You may need to drink a little more when you exercise, since you lose water through sweat and evaporation. Remember sufficient water intake is good, natural health insurance.

Drink Pure, Clean Water

If anti-aging is your goal, make sure that the water you drink is clean and pure. Most municipal water supplies contain contaminants and are heavily chlorinated and fluoridated. Some cities even add calcium hydroxide or other alkalinizing substances to alter the water's pH and prevent the corrosion of pipes. In addition, water pipes that contain copper or lead are linked to hypertension and other more serious conditions.

Purified water can be purchased at many stores, though most people don't realize that some bottled water is no better than tap water. Consider investing in a water-purification system that will consistently maintain the purity of your drinking water. This is ultimately more economical than buying bottled water — and the quality is usually better as well.

● ●

Safety and Precautions: Drinking too much water (over 100 ounces) can be harmful, as excess fluid consumption can stress the kidneys and digestive system. This is especially true if you have diabetes or hypertension, since these conditions can leave the kidneys in a weakened state.

Dosage and Timing: Hydrate your body with 64-80 ounces (eight to 10 eight-ounce glasses) of water spaced evenly throughout the day. Drink an additional four to six ounces every 15 minutes during workouts.

Other Nutritional Supplements to Consider

Many other supplements can substantially slow the aging process. However, these are beyond the scope of this book. Since not all nutritional requirements are satisfied by the LCAA Diet, we recommend the following supplements in addition to the ones described up until this point: macrominerals, including calcium, magnesium and potassium; a good source of dietary fiber (psyllium), essential fatty acids (see Chapter 7), and a broad spectrum multi vitamin-mineral formula.

 Hot Tip: Fiber is best taken in between meals, while vitamins, minerals and essential fatty acids are best taken with meals.

Table 8-1

LCAA Supplements

- A broad spectrum antioxidant formula, complete with vitamins A, C, and E, and beta carotene

- A macro-mineral formula, complete with calcium, magnesium and potassium

- Alpha lipoic acid — 100 - 600 mg per day

- Chromium (as picolinate or polynicotinate) — 400 - 600 mcg per day
- Vanadate (as vanadyl sulfate) — 50 - 150 mcg per day
- Gymnema sylvestre — Since potencies vary from product to product, it is best to follow dosage instructions on the label.

Plus these supplements to support mitochondrial function and encourage ketosis:

- Coconut oil — 2-4 tablespoons per day (this if for the medium chain triglyceride, MCT, content)
- CoQ10 — 150 mg per day
- Carnitine (or acetyl-l-carnitine, ALC) — 1,500-3,000 mg per day

And, of course:

- Exercise — daily
- Plenty of purified water
- Plenty of fish or an EFA supplement
- Lots of high-fiber, low-carbohydrate dark-green leafy vegetables (or a fiber supplement such as psyllium husk powder)

Chapter 9
Metformin
One of The Most Important
Life-Extending Supplements ... Is a Drug

O ne supplement that has demonstrated important benefits against insulin resistance is not a nutrient but a "smart drug." It's called *metformin*, and according to Ward Dean, M.D., co-author of *Smart Drugs and Nutrients,* it may be the "most effective and under-appreciated life extension drug" available.[194]

Recently introduced in the United States for the treatment of type II diabetes, *metformin* works by restoring insulin sensitivity to the cells. In this way, its actions are similar to vanadyl sulfate, with a stronger, more predictable action. Unlike other diabetic medications, which force increased insulin production (eventually destroying the pancreas), metformin works with the body by increasing the sensitivity of peripheral tissues to the effects of insulin.

> **Metformin ... may be the "most effective and under-appreciated life extension drug" available**
> **— Ward Dean, M.D.**

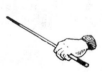

Metformin is chemically related to *phenformin*, an anti-diabetic drug that was discontinued in the United States in 1976 after a number of deaths were reported of diabetic patients. While the drug was safe for most diabetics, it was sometimes erroneously prescribed to patients with compromised liver and kidney function.

Metformin, a newer, less potent but much safer drug, carries many of the same health benefits as phenformin. According to Vladimir Dilman, M.D., co-author of *The Neuroendocrine Theory of Aging and Degenerative Disease,* these benefits include lower blood cholesterol, triglycerides and beta lipo-proteins, reduced development of atherosclerosis, reduced insulin levels, increased hypothalamo-pituitary sensitivity (declines with age), improved cellular immunity, reduced incidence of chemically induced cancer in rats, reduced growth of some tumors and enhanced action of certain anticancer medications. Most significantly, phenformin (and presumably metformin) increased the life span of laboratory animals.

According to Dr. Dean, most adults suffer from "subclinical" diabetes. He recommends the drug to all of his life-extension patients over the age of 40. However, he does note that one "potential side effect in long term users of metformin, is that it may cause malabsorption of vitamin B12." Dean goes on to recommend that "anyone taking metformin should also supplement their diet liberally with vitamin B12."[195]

Safety and Precautions: Because information regarding the use of metformin in the absence of carbohydrates is limited, we cannot recommend taking metformin with the LCAA Diet. While it may work well with the LGI Diet, the use of this drug should be carefully monitored by a licensed physician.

Dosage and Timing: Metformin is usually prescribed at a dosage of 500 mg taken twice a day, with meals.

Website: Please check our web site at www.smart-publications.com. You will find information on how to order pharmaceutical products by mail from overseas (for better selection and to save money), pointers on finding a suitable physician and a subscription button for our free e-newsletter.

Chapter 10
Exercise as a Fountain of Youth

Exercise can truly be considered a Fountain of Youth. The many health benefits of regular exercise range from increased strength and stamina to enhanced health and well being, and its anti-aging aspects are undeniable. Studies show that exercise can reduce insulin resistance, improve glucose tolerance, reduce body fat, enhance lean body mass, lower blood pressure, improve oxygen uptake, slow resting heart rate, reduce total cholesterol and triglycerides, raise HDL ("good") cholesterol and much more. Remarkably, physical exercise can even reverse coronary heart disease and reduce the risk of all-cause death![196]

Inactivity Is Risky

Most people are aware of the importance of exercise, but they just don't seem to get around to it. Yet the avoidance of exercise carries a heavy price tag. According to a joint statement from the American College of Sports Medicine and the Center for Disease Control and Prevention in Atlanta, an estimated 250,000 U.S. deaths a year are related to physical inactivity.[197]

Some medical researchers blame a sedentary lifestyle for the development of major chronic diseases. Defined as long-lasting illnesses that develop and worsen over time, chronic diseases are also considered "poorly understood and resistant to a cure."[198] Among those that may be prevented with regular exercise are coronary heart disease (CHD), hypertension, stroke, osteoporosis, type II diabetes, obesity, certain types of cancer and depression.[199]

With the exception of osteoporosis, the diseases linked with a sedentary lifestyle are the same as those produced by insulin resistance (syndrome X). These diseases are on the rise: Between

1901 and 1980, the U.S. deaths due to all chronic illnesses combined rose from 46 percent to 81 percent.[200] Insulin control through diet and lifestyle changes can be instrumental in stopping this trend.

Prevention Is the Best Medicine

Insulin resistance and glucose intolerance may increase with age, but exercise can do much to prevent this decline, especially when started in our younger years. A study of members of the Japan Self-Defense Forces recently demonstrated this. All of the participants were in their 50s and had some degree of impaired glucose tolerance (IGT). When their past fitness records and current glucose tolerance were compared, it was found that those who were most physically fit in their 30s had the healthiest blood sugar levels in their 50s.[201]

It's Never too Late

Whatever your age, it's never too late to reap the benefits of exercise. A Yale University study proved this when it tested the effects of aerobic exercise on volunteers who were in their 70s. The elderly men and women were split into two groups: a physical training and a control group. Aerobic exercise consisted of four 60-minute minitrampoline sessions a week, while the controls followed a mild program of stretching and yoga. After four months, the physically active group exhibited substantial improvements in glucose tolerance, while the control group showed no changes. [202]

Exercise Reverses Syndrome X!

Evidence suggests that exercise can reverse all of the metabolic disturbances associated with syndrome X. Over the past two decades, regular exercise has been shown to reverse obesity, cardiovascular heart disease, type II diabetes and other conditions related to insulin resistance.[203] Clearly, physical activity has a profoundly positive effect on restoring insulin sensitivity.

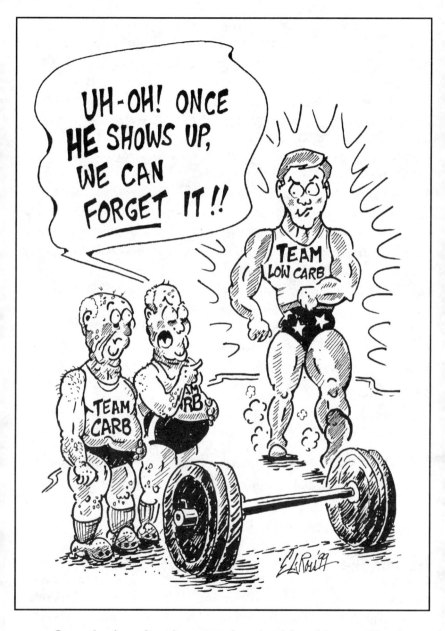

Over the last decade, several ground-breaking studies have verified that exercise reverses biological aging by improving insulin sensitivity in the skeletal muscles. One Swedish trial demonstrated that just one single exercise session improves insulin sensitivity in younger people. It also showed that middle-aged or older people can achieve the same benefit with just a few training sessions—and that these benefits can last for up to six days.[204] Think of it! Just two or three days of exercise can improve insulin sensitivity for nearly a week!

Improve Strength, Stamina and More—Exercise in Ketosis

As you begin the LCAA Diet, you may wonder whether you'll have the strength to exercise. That's because of the shift that takes place as the body switches from glucose to its own fat as its new fuel supply (see Chapter 4). By day three, you should notice a dramatic increase in your level of energy. This time frame is typical for people who are not taking mitochondrial nutrients and MCT. It may take far less time in supplementing individuals.

One four-week study on the effects of a low-carb diet (25 percent carbohydrate), found that the lower carbohydrate intake combined with exercise not only significantly improved the subjects' blood lipid profiles and reduced their body fat but provided plenty of energy for them to exercise.[205]

In a similar study of a very low carbohydrate ketogenic diet (5 percent carbohydrates, 45 percent protein, 50 percent fat), the researchers found that the diet increased the participants' total strength and stamina, improved their insulin levels and also increased their oxygen uptake.[206] Imagine having better strength and stamina while on the LCAA Diet!

Certain professional athletes, including some champion body builders, utilize an extreme ketosis diet to support their performance-enhancing goals. Many have adopted a program that includes absolutely no carbohydrates, with 40 percent of calories from protein and 60 percent from fat. These athletes expend a tremendous amount of energy during their workouts, yet find this diet provides all the energy they need. At the same time they are able to drastically reduce their body fat and increase their lean muscle mass.[207]

• •

 Safety and Precautions: A total deficit of carbohydrates would mean the total omission of nutrient-, enzyme- and fiber-rich vegetables, which are so important for health and longevity. Therefore, we don't recommend such a diet.

• •

Live Active, Live Longer

Two recent studies published in major medical journals confirmed what many of us already suspected: Exercise not only diminishes cardiovascular risk factors but significantly reduces death risk due to *all* causes.

The first, an extensive study of 16,936 Harvard alumni, followed their lifestyle habits and longevity. In the 12-to-16 year follow-up, 1,413 of the participants had died due to varying causes. The causes of death were 45 percent from cardiovascular disease, 32 percent from cancer, 13 percent from other natural causes and 10 percent from trauma. Curiously, regardless of the cause of death, exercise increased the life span in the 39 percent of those who were physically active.[208]

Another evaluation of 10,269 male Harvard alumni followed the effects of exercise, lifestyle and mortality. Again, the benefits of exercise were obvious. The men who engaged in moderately vigorous activity experienced a 41 percent reduced risk of heart disease death and a 23 percent reduced risk of death from all causes. The bottom line? Regardless of all other factors, physical activity was the most important factor for longevity.[209]

Begin Anti-Aging Exercise Today

Despite the well-known benefits of exercise, the majority of Americans still resist it. The U.S. Surgeon General and the American College of Sports Medicine estimate that fewer than 10 percent of Americans exercise at the recommended level and as many as 25 percent don't exercise at all!

Table 10-1
Some of the Benefits of Regular Exercise:

- Decrease body fat
- Improve glucose tolerance
- Improve mood and sense of well-being
- Increase HDL ("good") cholesterol
- Increase lean muscle mass
- Increase life expectancy
- Normalize blood pressure
- Reduce death risk due to all causes
- Reverse heart disease
- Reverse insulin resistance

In the not-so-distant past, physical activity was essential for life. In today's world, you can live much of your life exerting no more energy than walking from your home to your car and from your car to an elevator. Exercise is generally avoided because it is not perceived as a necessary component for life. A look at the scientific literature, however, suggests that it *is* necessary for life — at least for a longer, healthier one.

Choose Exercise That's Right for You

When beginning any exercise program, we strongly encourage you to find a physical activity you enjoy.* The key is to move continuously for about 30 minutes, three to five times a week. Keep in mind that if you haven't exercised in a while, this is a *goal,* it's not where you begin.

---

* **Note:** Sometimes it's *after* you've exercised that most of the enjoyment from physical activity comes — something to keep in mind while you're exercising.

Plan for Success

If you haven't exercised in a while, the thought of beginning an exercise routine may feel overwhelming. Some people read and watch television shows about exercise and are intimidated by what they think it entails. So start with something simple, like a brisk walk or bike ride (see Table 10-2). Then pace yourself as you gradually move toward your goal.

If you really want to get started, but find yourself resisting, we'd like to offer a practice that can positively cure your inability to *get up and go!*. Here's how it works:

On Day One, choose a form of movement that particularly suits you and do it for just one minute. On the following day, do it for two minutes. On the third day for three minutes and so on and so on. Do this, preferably, at the same time each day. You will find that after 21 days you will have created a powerful new habit. In addition, you will feel so good (including the confidence created by your success), that you won't want to give it up.

Table 10-2

Choose an Activity You Enjoy:

- Aerobics
- Bicycling
- Dancing
- Golfing
- Mini-Trampolining
- Skiing
- Swimming
- Yoga
- Walking
- Weight training

Hot tip: If you are using this technique, restrict yourself to the one, two and three, etc., minutes of exercise on each successive day. You will want to do more, and it is that experience of wanting more that we want to encourage. You'll soon find yourself looking forward to more exercise each day.

Two Great Exercises for a Lifetime of Fitness

If you can't decide on the best exercise(s) for you, we recommend you try a combination of walking and resistance (weight) training. Combined, these exercises provide an excellent balance of cardiovascular and strength-building benefits that can keep you looking and feeling youthful for a lifetime.

Walking provides a cardiovascular workout that improves circulation throughout your body, while also stimulating your large muscle groups. When you walk at a healthy, moderate pace, oxygen circulates to every cell of your body and, in the process, does you a world of good.

Simple Tips for a Successful Walking Program

- Purchase a good pair of walking shoes. Remember to break them in by wearing them around the house for a few hours before your first walk.

- Wear loose, comfortable clothing, such as cotton-based material that feels good against your skin. If you're in a cold climate, add layers that you can shed.

- Look for a safe and pleasant path, and steer clear of busy traffic areas. Instead, choose a scenic route with interesting vistas.

- To build up your intensity, pump your arms in opposite synchrony with your legs.

- Walk tall and with purpose. Think about how fabulous this exercise is for your body and mind.

- After your walk, cool down by stretching to improve your flexibility and allow your body to return to its resting state.

Strength Training for Strong Muscles and Bones

As we age, our muscles tend to atrophy from lack of exercise. Strength training, or resistance training, can prevent this wasting effect by keeping muscles strong and fit. It can even build new bone and muscle tissue. In mid-1999, the American College of Sports Medicine (ACSM) revised its fitness guidelines for people over 50, stating that strength training is the only exercise that can substantially slow and reverse age-related physiological declines such as bone and muscle tissue loss. ACSM recommends two to three weight training sessions per week, with special attention to the muscles of the arms, legs, shoulders and torso.[210]

To learn more about strength training programs, contact your local health club. Or use simple, inexpensive barbells right at home. You can use long bars to exercise both arms together and smaller dumbbells for single-arm exercises. Use weights that offer enough resistance for up to 15 repetitions per set before the muscles feel fatigued.

• •

Safety and Precautions: While getting enough exercise is important, it is equally important that you pace yourself. Too much exercise can increase free radical production and put you at risk for injuries. Do not be a weekend warrior, with sporadic, rigorous exercise. Instead, aim for moderate activities to which you can commit on a regular basis.

"Dosage and Timing": Choose one or several physical activities you enjoy and gradually work up to 30 minutes of continuous movement three to five times a week. Create an exercise regimen for yourself, for example, Monday, Wednesday and Friday mornings or afternoons. Once you reach your exercise goal, you may want to increase your workout time or change your exercise routine for variety.

Hot Tip: There are many excellent exercise programs available on television and video tape. Most of these can turn your living room or bedroom into a fine home gym.

Ask your mate or a friend to join you as an exercise buddy. For many, the mutual support works best for continued motivation. Dancing is a great aerobic exercise that can be extremely fun with a partner.

Chapter 11
The Complete LCAA Lifestyle

Investing in Your Most Valuable Asset

In this fast-paced world, many find it difficult to care for their own health. People in business are usually on some sort of deadline, without giving much thought to the deadline of life. All too often our most valuable asset, our health, is the most neglected. Yet when we buy a new car, we do everything necessary to maintain it.

By investing in this book, you have taken an important step toward caring for your physical body. In the coming weeks and months you will be investing your time, money and energy to produce powerful, positive changes in your life. While the complete LCAA lifestyle may not prevent old age, it certainly can control the usual effects of aging and disease by controlling your insulin and blood sugar levels. We suggest that you begin with either the Low Glycemic Index Diet or Low-Carb Anti-Aging Diet. Then improve your results with the addition of superfoods, healthy fats, nutritional supplements, pure water and regular exercise. For those serious about life extension, and who are over 40, we recommend using metformin under the guidance of a physician.

Use the Low Glycemic Index Diet to Your Advantage

If the ketosis level of carbohydrate consumption is not a comfortable program for you, we encourage you to follow the Low Glycemic Index Diet. This approach still reduces blood sugar and insulin levels, and allows you to gradually achieve similar results as with the Low-Carb Anti-Aging Diet. You may also opt to begin with the LGI Diet and transition to the LCAA Diet.

Follow the LCAA Diet for Faster Results

If safe, rapid weight loss is a part of your anti-aging goal, there is no better way than with the LCAA Diet. Studies have confirmed the long term safety of ketosis and low-carbohydrate eating , many of which are included in this book.

Find Your Own Best Carbohydrate Level

The amount of carbohydrates it takes to stay in ketosis varies for everyone. Get into ketosis by consuming just 10 to 20 grams of carbohydrate for the first two days. Then, by Day Three begin consuming a maximum of 30 carbohydrates per day, which is the amount that works best for most people. Once you have reached the deepest state of ketosis, we encourage you to experiment with small carbohydrate increases of just a few carbs per day (preferably by eating fresh, non-starchy vegetables). This is the best test of how many carbohydrates you can consume and still maintain ketosis.

Some people can eat as many 60 carbohydrates and remain in the deep state of ketosis (purple on the Ketostix®). Others must keep their carbohydrate intake at around 30, or sometimes even drop to 20 to achieve the desired effect. Your personal best carbohydrate level is the one that works best for you, so experiment until you reach a level that's right for you.

As we have said before, we do not recommend keeping your body in deep ketosis for long periods of time (such as weeks). Plus, very mild ketosis is easier to achieve and is sufficient to accomplish your goals of weight loss and health enhancement.

Mild ketosis is actually a state of metabolic **balance**, because both carbohydrate and fat metabolisms are active simultaneously. Ketosis is necessary because carbohydrate metabolism has priority

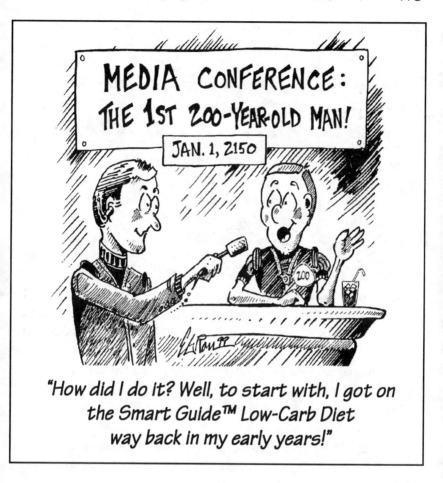

"How did I do it? Well, to start with, I got on the Smart Guide™ Low-Carb Diet way back in my early years!"

status and fat metabolism secondary (back-up) status. So you have both metabolisms only when carbohydrate metabolism is insufficient to meet energy needs and some fat burning is induced. So the concept we propose is one of duality in energy production: To be optimized in health, you want both pathways active **at the same time**.

Focus on Low-Carb Superfoods

Low-Carb superfoods such as soy (tofu), whey protein concentrate (WPC), and fresh low starch vegetables are major allies on the LCAA Diet. The regular consumption of these wholesome foods can make a tremendous difference in your health by helping to prevent disease, improve immunity, promote bone density, balance hormone levels and increase your vitality. Be sure to eat some of these every day. If you need help getting them into your diet, we recommend *The Low-Carb Anti-Aging Diet Cookbook*, available through Smart Publications.

● ●

Website: Please check our web site at www.smart-publications.com. You will find information on how to order *The Low-Carb Anti-Aging Diet Cookbook* and other books and a subscription button for our free e-newsletter.

● ●

Focus on Healthy Fats that Make You Lean

As you follow the LCAA Diet, you will find that most fats are your friends. Health-promoting fats such as fish, flax and coconut oils help to induce and maintain ketosis, protect against disease, reduce body fat, satiate appetite and boost your metabolism. We suggest you eat plenty of fatty fish (such as salmon) or take about 6 grams of fish oil per day.

If you don't want to eat fish or fish oil, take flax seed or about one tablespoon of flax oil per day. Additionally take one tablespoon of coconut oil each day. Also remember to avoid margarine, shortening such as Crisco® and other processed, trans, oxidized or altered fats.

Take Your Anti-Aging Supplements

While many supplements are touted as "anti-aging," we have focused on those that directly influence insulin resistance. With syndrome X, consistently high levels of insulin and glucose can lead to the breakdown of major physiological systems. These can, however, be controlled with adequate antioxidant intake. Vitamins

C, E, and beta carotene, and selenium provide superior anti-aging protection, as they help to protect against free-radical, AGEs and cross-link damage. Alpha lipoic acid (ALA), another important antioxidant, can actually reverse and prevent some of the damage caused by high insulin levels.

In addition to antioxidants, the trace minerals chromium and vanadium are an excellent adjunct to the LCAA Diet. Combined, they can produce balanced glucose and insulin levels and even help to restore insulin sensitivity. For best results, take them together with an herbal extract of Gymnema sylvestre. And remember to drink plenty of pure water!

Become Physically Active

While exercise is not a required part of this program, it is one anti-aging strategy that really works. Regular physical activity steadily increases the body's insulin sensitivity, glucose tolerance, and even reduces the risk of all-cause death. Once you've identified the best activity for you, choose to make it a regular part of your healthy lifestyle. We recommend an exercise goal of at least 30 minutes of continuous movement three to five times per week. Just remember to pace yourself as you gradually move toward your exercise goal.

Establish a Routine to Control Insulin and Aging for a Lifetime

The complete LCAA lifestyle will work best if you plan and follow a simple, daily anti-aging routine. Breakfast and a brisk morning walk can start your day and put you right on track. Keep plenty of low-carb foods on hand that you enjoy. Place your nutritional supplements where you will easily see them and remember to take them daily.

The Ultimate Gift

While the psychological aspects of anti-aging are beyond the scope of this book, we do acknowledge that these play a major role in anti-aging and longevity. In short, be sure to take care of your emotional well being.

Do what you can to manage stress and get enough sleep. If you set goals, keep them realistic. Acknowledge your successes and take time every day to appreciate some aspects of your life, such as by keeping a gratitude journal. Finally, find the time to admire nature, play with a child, laugh at a joke or listen to a friend. You will be amazed at how much more you enjoy this diet, your work and the all of the other aspects of your life. Life, after all, is the ultimate gift.

Resources

Smart Publications Web Site
www.smart-publications.com

Information on Glycemic Index
Glycemic Research Institute
601 Pennsylvania Ave., N.W.
Washington, D.C. 20004.
(202) 434-8270

Whey and Soy Protein Concentrates
Next Proteins™
P.O. Box 2469
Carlsbad, Calif. 92018
(800)GOT-NEXT

Atkins Nutritionals, Inc.
Atkins has shakes, ketosis sticks, bake mixes, and other valuable resources.
185 Oser Ave.
Hauppauge, N. Y. 11788
(800) 628-5467

For Organic Produce
CSA: Community-Supported Agriculture. Groups that contract area farmers who agree to grow organic produce.
Robyn Van En Center for CSA Resources
(717) 264-4141 ext. 3247 or

Biodynamic Farming and Gardening Association
(800) 516-7797.

For Organic Coconut Oil

Spectrum Naturals
Petaluma, Calif.
(800) 995 2705
www.spectrumnaturals.com

For Organic Meats, Eggs and Dairy Products

Organic Valley
La Farge, WI
(888) 444-6455 voice
www.organicvalley.com

References

1   Zavoroni, I. et al. Risk factors for coronary artery disease in healthy persons with hyperin-sulinemia and normal glucose tolerance. *The New England Journal of Medicine*. 1989; 320:702-6.

2   DeFronzo, R, Ferrannini, E. Insulin Resistance - a multifaceted syndrome responsible for NIDDM, obesity, hypertension, dyslipidemia, and atherosclerotic cardiovascular disease, *Diabetes Care*. 1991; 14(3):173-94.

3   Schoen RE, et al. Increased blood glucose and insulin, body size, and incident colorectal cancer. *J Natl Cancer Inst*. 1999;91(13):1147-1154.

4   Reaven, G. Role of insulin resistance in human disease. *Diabetes*. 1988;37, 1595-1607.

5   Reaven, G. Syndrome X. *Clinical Diabetes*. 1994;3-4, 32-52.

6   Reaven, G. Syndrome X: 6 years later. *J Int Med Suppl*. 1994;736:13-22.

7   McCarty MF. Enhancing central and peripheral insulin activity as a strategy for the treat-ment of endogenous depression. *Med Hypotheses*. 1994;43(4):247-252.

8   Muller DC, et al. The effect of age on insulin resistance and secretion: a review. *Semin Nephrol*. 1996.16(4):289-298.

9   Iozzo P, et al. Independent influence of age on basal insulin secretion in nondiabetic humans. European Group for the Study of Insulin Resistance. *J Clin Endocrinol Metab*. 1999;84(3):863-868.

10 Dilman, V, Dean.,W. *The Neuroendocrine Theory of Aging and Degenerative Disease*. Pensacola, FL: The Center for Bio-Gerontology, 1992.

11 Mooradian AD, Thurman, JE. Glucotoxicity. *Clinics in Geriatric Med*.1999;15(2)255-263.

12 Wexler BC, Comparative aspects of hyperadrenocortiscism and aging. In:*Hypothalamus, Pituitary and Aging* by Everitt AV, Burgess, JA (Eds.)Charles C Thomas, Springfield, MA; 1976: 333-361.

13 Carantoni M, et al. Relationships between fasting plasma insulin, anthropometrics, and metabolic parameters in a very old healthy population. Associazone Medica Sabin. *Metabolism*. 1998;47(5):535-40.

14 Stoll BA. Western diet, early puberty, and breast cancer risk. *Breast Cancer Res Trat*. 1998;49(3):187-193.

15 Slattery ML, et al. Dietary sugar and colon cancer. *Cancer Epidemiol Biomarkers Prev*. 1997;6(9):677-685.

16 DeFronzo, R, Ferrannini, E. Insulin Resistance - a multifaceted syndrome responsible for NIDDM, obesity, hypertension, dyslipidemia, and atherosclerotic cardiovascular disease, *Diabetes Care*. 1991; 14(3):173-94.

17 Zavoroni, I. et al.Risk factors for coronary artery disease in healthy persons with hyperin-sulinemia and normal glucose tolerance. *The New England Journal of Medicine*. 1989;320:702-6.

18 Reaven, G. Syndrome X. *Clinical Diabetes*. 1994;3-4, 32-52.

19 Endre, T. Insulin resistance is coupled to low physical fitness in normotensive men with a family history of hypertension. *Journal of Hypertension*. 1994; 12, 81-88.

20 Dilman, V, Dean.,W. *The Neuroendocrine Theory of Aging and Degenerative Disease*. Pensacola, FL: The Center for Bio-Gerontology, 1992.

21 Dilman, V, Dean.,W. *The Neuroendocrine Theory of Aging and Degenerative Disease*. Pensacola, FL: The Center for Bio-Gerontology, 1992.

22   Ibid.

23   Everson SA, et al. Weight gain and the risk of developing insulin resistance syndrome. *Diabetes Care.* 1998;21(10):1637-1643.

24   Silver F, Brecciaroli D, Argentati F, Cervini C. Serum levels of insulin in overweight patients with osteoarthritis of the knee. *J Rheumatol.* 1994;21(10):1899-1902.

25   Smythe HA. Osteoarthritis, insulin and bone density. *J Rheumatol.* 1987;14:91-93.

26   American Heart Association, 1997

27   Lempianen P, et al. Insulin resistance syndrome predicts coronary heart disease events in elderly nondiabetic men.*Circulation.* 1999;100(2):123-128.

28   Pyorala M, et al. Hyperinsulinemia predicts coronary heart disease risk in healthy middle-aged men: the 22-year follow-up results in the Finnish Helsinki Policeman Study. *Circulation.* 1998;4;98(5): 398-404.

29   Fontbonne A, et al. Body fat distribution and coronary heart disease mortality in subjects with impaired glucose tolerance or diabetes mellitus: the Paris Prospective Study, 15-year follow-up. *Diabetologia.* 1992;35 (5):464-8.

30   Zavoroni I. et al. Risk factors for coronary artery disease in healthy persons with hyperinsulinemia and normal glucose tolerance. *The New England Journal of Medicine.* 1989;320:702-6.

31   DeFronzo R, Ferrannini E. Insulin Resistance - a multifaceted syndrome responsible for NIDDM, obesity, hypertension, dyslipidemia, and atherosclerotic cardiovascular disease, *Diabetes Care.* 1991; 14(3):173-94.

32   Zimlichman R, et al. Hyperinsulinemia induces myocardial infarctions and arteriolar medial hypertrophy in spontaneously hypertensive rats. *Am J Hypertens.* 1997;10(6):646-653.

33   Festa A, et al. Relative contribution of insulin and its precursors to fibrinogen and PAI-1 in a large population with different states of glucose tolerance. The Insulin Resistance Atherosclerosis Study (IRAS). *Arterioscler Thromb Vasc Biol.* 1999;19(3):562-568.

34   Lazarus R, et al. Impaired ventilatory function and elevated insulin levels in nondiabetic males: the Normative Aging Study.*Eur Respir J.* 1998;12(3):635-640.

35   American Diabetes Association, 1997.

36   Bierhaus A, et al. AGEs and their interaction with AGE-receptors in vascular disease and diabetes mellitus. I. The AGE concept. *Cardiovasc Res.*1998;37(3):586-600.

37   Kappel M, et al. Immunological effects of a hyperinsulinaemic euglycaemic insulin clamp in healthy males. *Scan J Immunol.* 1998;47(4):363-368.

38   Schoen RE, et al. Increased blood glucose and insulin, body size, and incident colorectal cancer. *J Natl Cancer Inst.* 1999;91(13):1147-1154.

39   Nagamani M, Stuart CA. Specific binding and growth-promoting activity of insulin in endometrial cancer cells in culture. *Am J Obstet Gynecol.* 1998;179(1):6-12.

40   Dechenes CJ, et al. Human aging is associated with parallel reductions in insulin and amylin release. *Am J Phsiol.* 1998;275(5 Pt 1):E785-791.

41   Moore MA, Park CB, Tsuda H. Implications of the hyperinsulinaemia-diabetes-cancer link for preventative efforts. *Eur J Cancer Prev.* 1998; (2):89-107.

42   Stoll BA. Western diet, early puberty, and breast cancer risk. *Breast Cancer Res Treat.* 1998;49(3):187-193.

43   Eades MR, Eades MD. *Protein Power* New York, NY: Bantam Books, 1996.

44   Eaton SB, Konner M. Paleolithic nutrition. *New Engl J of Med.* 1985;312 (5):283-289.

45   Slattery ML, et al. Dietary sugar and colon cancer. *Cancer Epidemiol Biomarkers Prev.* 1997;6(9):677-685.

46   Burley VJ. Sugar consumption and cancers of the digestive tract. *Eur J Cancer*

*Prev.*1997;6(5):422-434.

47 D Stafani E, et al. Dietary sugar and lung cancer: a case-control study in Uruguay. *Nutr Cancer.* 1998;31(2):132-137.

48 Slattery ML, et al. Dietary sugar and colon cancer. *Cancer Epidemiol Biomarkers Prev.* 1997;6(9):677-685.

49 Mooradian AD, Thurman, JE. Glucotoxicity. *Clinics in Geriatric Med.*1999;15(2)255-263.

50 Mooradian AD, Thurman, JE. Glucotoxicity - potential mechanisms. *Clinics in Geriatric Med.* 1999; 15(2):255-263.

51 Balkau B, et al. High blood glucose concentration is a risk factor for mortality in middle-aged nondiabetic men. 20-year follow-up in the Whitehall Study, the Paris Prospective Study, and the Helsinki Policemen Study. *Diabetes Care.* 1998;21(3):360-367.

52 Keeton, K. *Longevity: the science of staying young* . New York, NY: Viking Penguin; 1992.

53 Mizutarii K, Photo-enhanced modification of human skin elastin in actinic elastosis. *J Invest Dermatol.* 1997;108(5):797-802.

54 Mooradian AD, Thurman, JE. Glucotoxicity - potential mechanisms. *Clinics in Geriatric Med.* 1999; 15(2):255-263.

55 Odetti P, et al. Good glycaemic control reduces oxidation and glycation end-products in collagen of diabetic rats. *Diabetologia.* 1996;39(12):1440-1447.

56 Lyons TJ, et al. Decrease in skin collagen glycation with improved glycemic control in patients with insulin-dependent diabetes mellitus. *J Clin Invest.* 1991;87(6):1910-1915.

57 Wolever TM, et al. Beneficial effect of low-glycemic index diet in overweight NIDDM subjects. *Diabetes Care.* 1992;15(4):562-564.

58 Odetti P, et al. Good glycaemic control reduce oxidation and glycation end-products in collagen of diabetic rats. *Diabetologia.* 1996;39(12):1440-1447.

59 Jenkins, D, Wolever, T. Glycemic index of foods: a physiologic basis for carbohydrate exchange. *The American Journal of Clinical Nutrition.* 1981; 34:362-366.

60 Podell, R.*The G-Index Diet..* New York, NY: Warner Books Inc.; 1993.

61 Ludwig DS, et al. High glycemic index foods, overeating, and obesity. *Pediatrics.* 1999;103(3):E26.

62 Franceshi S, et al. Food groups and risk of colorectal cancer in Italy. *Int J Cancer.* 1997;72(1):56-61.

63 Ibid.

64 Levi B, Werman MJ. Long-term fructose consumption accelerates glycation and several age-related variables in male rats. *J Nutr.* 1998;128(9):1442-1449.

65 de Wees Allen, A. The Glycemic Index: glycemic impact of food. http://www.anndeweesallen.com/dal-gly2.htm

66 Odetti P, et al. Good glycaemic control reduces oxidation and glycation end-products in collagen of diabetic rats. *Diabetologia.* 1996;39(12):1440-1447.

67 Richard, D. *Stevia Rebaudiana: Nature's Sweet Secret.* Bloomingdale, Illinois: Blue Heron Press, 1996.

68 McArdle WD, Katch FI, Katch VL. *Exercise Physiology: Energy, Nutrition and Human Performance.* Philadelphia, PA: Lea & Ferbiger; 1986.

69 Dilman, V, Dean.,W. *The Neuroendocrine Theory of Aging and Degenerative Disease.* Pensacola, FL: The Center for Bio-Gerontology, 1992.

70 Atkins, RC. *Dr. Atkins' New Diet Revolution.* New York, NY: M. Evans and Company , Inc.; 1992.

71 Eaton SB, Konner, M. Paleolithic nutrition. *New Engl J of Med.* 1985;312 (5):283-289.

72 Atkins, RC. *Dr. Atkins' New Diet Revolution*. New York, NY: M. Evans and Company, Inc.; 1992.

73 Ibid.

74 Carroll J, Koenigsberger D. The ketogenic diet: a practical guide for caregivers. *J Am Diet Assoc*. 1998;98(3):316-321.

75 Nebeling, LC. Implementing a ketogenic diet based on medium-chain triglyceride oil in pediatric patients with cancer. *J Am Diet Assoc*. 1995;95:693-697.

76 Ibid.

77 Magee BA, et al. The inhibition of malignant cell growth by ketone bodies. *Aust J Exp Biol Med Sci*.1979. 57(5):529-239.

78 Phinney SD, et al. The human metabolic response to chronic ketosis without caloric restriction: physical and biochemical adaptation.*Metabolism*.1983;32(8):757-768.

79 Willi SM, et al. The effects of a high-protein, low-fat, ketogenic diet on adolescents with morbid obesity: body composition, blood chemistries, and sleep abnormalities. *Pediatrics*. 1998;101(1):61-67.

80 Ibid.

81 Golay A, et al. Weight-loss with low or high carbohydrate diet?*Int J Obes Relat Metab Disord*. 1996;20(12):1067-1072

82 Evans E, et al. The absence of undesirable changes during consumption of the Low-Carbohydrate diet. *Nutr Metabol*. 1974;17:360-367.

83 Benoit, F. et al. Changes in body composition during weight reduction in obesity. *Archives of Internal Medicine;* 1965;63 (4):604-612.

84 Blackburn G, et al. Preservation of the physiological responses in a protein sparing modified fast. *Cent Nut Res.*, NEDH and the Dept Nut & Fd Sci., MIT, Boston Mass.

85 Johnson WA, Weinger, MW. Protective effects of ketogenic diets on signs of hypoglycemia. *Diabetes*.1978;27(11):1087-1091.

86 Spring B, et al. Psychobiological effects of carbohydrates. *J Clin Psychiatry*. 1989;50(5):27-33

87 Spring B. et al Effects of protein and carbohydrate meals on mood and performance: interaction with sex and age. *J Psychiatry Res*. 1983;17(2):155-167.

88 Adlercreutz H, Mazur W. Phyto-oestrogens and Western disease. *Annals of Med*. 1997;29:95-120.

89 Anderson JB, Garner SC. Phytoestrogens and human function. *Nutr Today*. 1997;32(6):232-9

90 Ibid

91 Kurzer MS, Zu X. Dietary phytoestrogens. *Annu Rev Nutr*. 1997;17:353--381.

92 Ham, JO, et al. Endocrinological response to soy protein and fiber in mildly hypercholesterolemic men. *Nutr Res*. 1993;13:873-874.

93 Sanchez A, Hubbard RW. Plasma amino acids and the insulin/glucagon ratio as an explanation of the dietary protein modulation of atherosclerosis. *Med Hypothesis*. 1991;35:324-329.

94 Sirtori CR, et al. Soy bean-protein diet in the treatment of type-II hyperliprotemia. *Lancet*. 1977;1:275-277.

95 Anderson, JB, Garner SC. Phytoestrogens and human function. *Nutr. Today*. 1997;32(6):232-239.

96 Nestel PJ,et al. Soy isoflavones improve systemic arterial compliance but not plasma lipids in menopausal and perimenopausal women. *Arterioscler Thromb Vasc Biol*. 1997; 17(12):3392-3398.

97 Coward L, et al. Genistein, daidzein, and their beta-glycoside conjugates: anti tumor isoflavones in soybean foods from American and Asian diets. *J Agric Food Chem.* 1993;41:1961-1967.

98 Lu, LW, et al. Effects of soya consumption for one mother on steroid hormones in pre-menopausal women: implications for breast cancer risk reduction. *Cancer Epidemiol Biomarkers Prev.* 1996;5:63-70.

99 Kyle, E. et al. Genistein-induced apoptosis of prostate cancer cells is preceded by a specific decrease in focal adhesion kinase activity. *MOl Pharmacol.* 1997;51 (2):193-200.

100 Arjmandi BH, et al. Dietary soybean protein prevents bone loss in an ovariectomized rat model of osteoporosis. *J Nutr.* 1996;126:161-167.

101 Dalias FS, et al. Dietary soy supplementation increases vaginal cytology maturation index and bone mineral content in postmenopausal women. *Second International Symposium on the Role of Soy in Preventing and Treating Chronic Disease.* (Brussels, Belgium, 1996).

102 Kurzer MS, Zu X. Dietary phytoestrogens. *Annu Rev Nutr.* 1997;17:353--381.

103 Guyton AC. Protein Metabolism. In Textbook of Medical Physiology 8th ed. Philadelphia (PA): W.B. Saunders; 1991.

104 Boirie Y, et al. Slow and fast dietary proteins differently modulate postprandial protein accretion. *Porc Nautl Acad Sci.* 1997;94:14930-14935.

105 Renner E. Milk Protein. In: Milk and Dairy Products in Human Nutrition. Munich: Volksvirtschaftlicher Verlag; 1983.

106 Preliminary study conducted at the University of Nebraska, Omaha. 1996, 1997. Courtesy of Next Nutrition.

107 Brink, W.The wonders of whey.*Life Extension.* 1999;5(5):35-39.

108 Sadler, R. The benefits of dietary whey protein concentrate on the immune response and health. *S Afr J Dairy Sci.* 1992;24 (2):53-59.

109 Ibid.

110 Kennedy RS, et al. The use of whey protein concentrate in the treatment of patients with metastic carcinoma: A phase I-II clinical study. *Anticancer Res.* 1995;15:2643-2650.

111 McIntosh GH, et al. Dairy proteins protect against dimethylhydrazine-induced intestinal cancers in rats. *J Nutr.* 1995;125:809-816.

112 Chmiel JF et al. *Proceedings of the Second International Whey Conference, IIDF/FIL 9804,* 1997:310-325.

113 Nagaoka S, et al. Comparative studies on the serum cholesterol lowering action of whey protein and soybean protein in rats. *Bioscience, Biotech, and Biochem.* 1992;56(9):1484-1485.

114 Sautier C, et al. Effects of whey protein, casein, soya-bean and sunflower proteins on the serum, tissue, and faecal steroids in rats. *J Nutr.* 1983;49:313-318.

115 Takada Y, et al. Whey protein stimulates the proliferation and differentiation of osteoblastic MC3T3 cells. *Biochem and Biophys Res Com.* 1996;223:445-449.

116 Franceshi S, et al. Food groups and risk of colorectal cancer in Italy. *Int J Cancer.* 1997;72(1):56-61.

117 Weil, A. The power of produce. *Self Healing.* 1999;7:1-7.

118 Steinmetz KA, Potter JD. Vegetables, fruit, and cancer. II. Mechanisms. *Cancer Causes Control.* 1991;2(6):427-442.

119 Ibid.

120 Michnovicz JJ, Bradlow HL. Altered estrogen metabolism and excretion in humans following consumption of indole-3-carbinol. *Nutrition and Cancer.* 1991;16:59-66.

121 No author. I3C the tamoxifen substitute. *Life Extension.* 1999;10:28-34.

122 Yochum L, et al. Dietary flavonoid intake and risk of cardiovascular disease in post-menopausal women. *Am J Epidemiol.* 1999;148(10):943-949.

123 Mazur W. Phytoestrogen content in foods. *Bailliere's Clin Endocrin and Metab.* 1998;12(4):729-743.

124 Koch HP, Lawson LD, eds. *Garlic -- The Science and Therapeutic Application of Allium sativum L. and Related Species.* 2nd ed. Baltimore, MD: Williams & Wilkins, 1996.

125 Tyler VE. *The Honest Herbal. 3rd edition.* Binghamton, NY: Pharmaceutical Press, 1993.

126 Ibid.

127 Oliver MF. It is more important to increase the intake of unsaturated fats than to decrease the intake of saturated fats:evidence from clinical trial relating to ischemic heart disease. *Am J Clin Nutr.* 1997;66(S):980S-986S.

128 Berry EM. Dietary fatty acids in the management of diabetes mellitus. *Am J Clin Nutr.* 1997;66(S):991S-997S.

129 Rose DP. Dietary fatty acids and cancer. *Am J Clin Nutr.* 1997;66(S):998S-1003S.

130 Coutatre, D. Anti-Fat Nutrients.San Francisco, CA: Pax Publishing; 1997.

131 Dean C. Fat fight.*Natural Health.*1999;6:98-141.

132 Dilman, V, Dean.,W. *The Neuroendocrine Theory of Aging and Degenerative Disease.* Pensacola, FL: The Center for Bio-Gerontology, 1992.

133 Atkins, RC. *Dr. Atkins' New Diet Revolution.* New York, NY: M. Evans & Company, Inc.,1992.

134 Erasmus, U. *Fats that Heal Fats that Kill.* Vancouver, Canada: Alive Books, 1993.

135 Lou J, et al. Dietary (n-3) polyunsaturated fatty acids improve adipocyte insulin action and glucose metabolism in insulin-resistant rats: relation to membrane fatty acids. *J Nutr.* 1996;126(8):1951-1058.

136 Borkman M, et al. Effects of fish oil supplementation on glucose and lipid metabolism in NIDDM. *Diabetes.* 1989;38(10):1314-1319.

137 Simopoulos AP. Omega-3 fatty acids in the prevention-management of cardiovascular disease. *Can J Physiol Pharmacol.* 1997;75(3):234-239.

138 Kromhout D, et al. Inverse relation between fish oil consumption and 20 year mortality from coronary heart disease. *N Engl J Med.* 1985;312:1205-1209.

139 Sedielin KN, et al. N-3 fatty acids in adipose tissue and coronary artery disease are inversely correlated. *Am J Clin Nutr.* 1992;55:1117-1119.

140 Hu FB, et al. Dietary intake of alpha-linolenic acid and risk of fatal ischemic heart disease among women. *Am J Clin Nutr.* 1999;69:890-897.

141 Whitaker J. Fish oil: a favorite therapy revisited.*Health & Healing.*1999; 9(7):4-6.

143 Cobias L, et al. Lipid, lipoprotein, and hemostatic effects of fish vs fish oil s-3 fatty acids in mildly hyperlipidemic males. *Am J Clin Nutr.* 1991;53:1201-1216.

144 Bao DQ, et al. Effects of dietary fish and weight reduction on ambulatory blood pressure in overweight hypertensives. *Hypertension.* 1998;32(4):710-717.

145 Allman MA, et al. Supplementation with flaxseed oil versus sunflower seed oil in healthy young men consuming a low fat diet: effects on platelet composition and function. *Eur J Clin Nutr.* 1995;49(3):169-178.

146 Kaunitz H. Medium chain triglycerides (MCT) in aging and arteriosclerosis. *Environ Pathol Toxicol Oncol.* 1986;6(3-4):115-121.

147 Peat, R. Coconut oil. *Townsend Letter for Doctors and Patients.*1995;143:152-156

148 Ibid.

149 Portillo MP, et al. Energy restriction with high-fat diet enriched with coconut oil gives high-

er UCP2 and lower white fat in rats. *Int J Obes Relat Metab Disord.* 1998;22(10):974-979.

150 Cox, C. Effects of coconut oil, butter, and safflower oil on lipids and lipo-proteins in persons with moderately elevated cholesterol levels. *J Lipid Res.* 1995;36:1787-1795.

151 Kaunitz H. Medium chain triglycerides (MCT) in aging and arteriosclerosis. *Environ Pathol Toxicol Oncol.* 1986;6(3-4):115-121.

152 Carroll J, Koenigsberger D. The ketogenic diet: a practical guide for caregivers. *J Am Diet Assoc.* 1998;98(3):316-321.

153 Nebeling, LC. Implementing a ketogenic diet based on medium-chain triglyceride oil in pediatric patients with cancer. *J Am Diet Assoc.* 1995;95:693-697.

154 Lev-Ran A. Mitogenic factors accelerate later-age diseases: insulin as a paradigm. *Mech Ageing Dev.* 1998;102(1):95-113.

155 Atkins, RC. *Dr. Atkins' New Diet Revolution.* New York, NY: M. Evans & Company, Inc.,1992.

156 Gordon S. The case for organic food. *New Age.* 1999;5:70-86.

157 Kromhout D, et al. Dietary saturated and trans-fatty acids and cholesterol and 25-year mortality from coronary heart disease: the Seven Countries Study. *Prev Med.* 1996;24(3):308-315.

158 Gillman MW, et al. Margarine intake and subsequent coronary heart disease in men. *Epidemiology.* 1997;8(2):122-123.

159 Awad AB, et al.trans-fatty acids in tumor development and the host survival. *J Natl Cancer Inst.*1981;67(1):189-192.

160 Otero O. Are trans-fatty acids a serious risk for disease.*Am J Clin Nutr.* 1997;66(S):1018S-1019S.

161 Deguine V, et al. Free radical depolymerization of hyaluronan by Maillard reaction products: role in liquefaction of aging vitreous. 1998;22(1):17-22

162 Ginter E. Cardiovascular disease prevention in Eastern Europe. *Nutrition.* 1998;14(5):452-457.

163 Fu MX, et al. Glycation, glycoxidation, and cross-linking of collagen by glucose...inhibition of late stages of Maillard reaction. *Diabetes.* 1994; 43(5):676-683.

164 Deguine, V. et al. Free radical depolymerization of hyaluronan by Maillard reaction products: role in liquefaction of aging vitreous. *Int J. Biol Macromol* 1998;22(1):17-22.

165 Booth AA, et al. In vitro kinetic studies of formation of antigenic advanced glycation end products (AGEs). Novel inhibition of post-Amadori glycation pathways. ... may prevent initial sugar attachment.*J Biol Chem.* 1997;272(9):5430-5437.

166 Kagan VE, et al., Dihydrolipoic acid—A universal antioxidant both in the membrane and in the aqueous phase. *Biochem Pharmacol* . 1992;44:1637-1649.

167 Corlett S. *Stabilized Rice Bran...Nutrition & Diabetes.* Winter Havens, FL: DRC Publications, Inc., 1997.

168 Estrada DE, et al. Stimulation of glucose uptake by the natural coenzyme alpha-lipoic acid/thioctic acid: participation of elements of the insulin signaling pathway. *Diabetes.* 1996;45(23):1798-1804.

169 Ziegler, D. et al. Treatment of symptomatic diabetic peripheral neuropathy with the antioxidant a-lipoic acid. The 3-week multicentre randomized controlled trial (Aladin Study). *Diabetologia.* 1995;38:1425-1433.

170 Kahler W, et al. Diabetes mellitus and free radical-associated disease. Results of adjuvent antioxidant supplementation. *A Gesamte Inn Med.* 1993;48:223-232.

171 Scholich H, et al. Antioxidant activity of dihydrolipoate against microsomal lipid peroxidation and its dependence on a-tocopherol. *Biochem Biophys Acta.* 1989;1001:256-261.

172 No author listed. Alpha lipoic acid. *Alt Med Rev.* 1998;3(4):308-311.

173 Gal EM. Reversal of selective toxicity of (-)-a-lipoic acid by thiamine in thiamin-deficient rats. *Nature* 1965;205:535

174 Mahdi GS. Chromium deficiency might contribute to insulin resistance, type 2 diabetes mellitus, dyslipidemia, and atherosclerosis.*Diabet. Med.* 1996;13(4):389-390.

175 Ibid.

176 Ravina A, et al. Clinical use of the trace element chromium (III) in the treatment of diabetes mellitus. *J Trace Elem Exp Med.* 1995;8:183-190.

177 Anderson RA, et al. Elevated intakes of supplemental chromium improve glucose and insulin variables in individuals with type 2 diabetes. *Diabetes.* 1997;46(11):1786-1791.

178 Kaats FR, et al. A randomized, double-masked, placebo-controlled study of the effects of chromium picolinate supplementation on body composition: a replication and extension of a previous study. *Curr Therap Res.* 1998;59(6):379-388.

179 Whitaker, J. Chromium toxicity: tempest in a teapot. *Health & healing.* 1999;9(8):1-4.

180 Badmaev V, et al. Vanadium: a review of its potential role in the fight against diabetes. *J Altern Complement Med.* 2999;5(3):273-291.

181 Reul BA, et al. Effects of vanadium complexes with organic ligands on glucose metabolism: a comparison study in diabetic rats. *Br J Pharmacol.* 1999;126(2):467-477.

182 Usman H, et al. Effects of chronic vanadate administration in the STZ-Induced diabetic rat. *Diabetes.* 1995;43:9-15

183 McNeill, J. Enhanced in vivo sensitivity of vanadyl-treated diabetic rats to insulin. *Canadian Journal of Physiology and Pharmacology* 1996. 68 (4):486-91.

184 Cam MC, et al. Partial preservation of pancreatic beta-cells by vanadium: evidence for long-term amelioration of diabetes. *Metabolism.* 1997;46(7):769-778.

185 Boden G, et al. Effects of vanadyl sulfate on carbohydrate and lipid metabolism in patients with non-insulin-dependent diabetes mellitus. *Metabolism.* 1996;45(9):1130-1135.

186 Cohen N, et al. Oral vanadyl sulfate improves hepatic and peripheral insulin sensitivity in patients with non-insulin-dependent diabetes mellitus. *J Clin Invest.* 1995;95(6):2501-2509.

187 Badmaev V, et al. Vanadium: a review of its potential role in the fight against diabetes. *J Altern Complement Med.* 2999;5(3):273-291.

188 Poucheret P, Verma S, Grynpas M, McNeill J. Vanadium and diabetes. *Mol. Cell. Biochem.* 1998;188(102):73-80.

189 Harland BF, Harden-Williams BA. Is vanadium of human nutritional importance yet? *J Am Diet Assoc.* 1994;94:891-894.

190 Baskaran K et al. Antidiabetic effect of a leaf extract from Gymnema sylvestre in non-insulin-dependent diabetes mellitus patients. *J Ethnopharmacol.* 1990;30:295-305.

191 Shanmugasundaram ERB, et al. Use of Gymnema sylvestre leaf extract in the control of blood glucose in insulin-dependent diabetes mellitus.*J Ethnopharmacol.* 1990;30:281-294.

192 Batmanghelidj, F. *Your Body's Many Cries for Water.* Falls Church, VA:Global Health Solutions, Inc., 1995.

193 Ibid.

194 Dean, W. Metformin, the most effective and under-appreciated life extension drug.*Vitamin Research Products.* November 1998;12 (9).

195 Ibid.

196 Suominen, H. Effects of physical training in middle-aged and elderly people. In: Komi, P.V. (Ed.), *Studies in Sports, Physical Education and Health* 11, University of Jyvaskyla, 1978.

197 Somer, E. Age-Proof Your Body, New York, NY: William Morrow & Co., 1998.

198 Powel, KE, et al. Physical activity and chronic diseases. *Am J Clin Nutr.* 1989;49:999-1006

199 Ibid.

200 Ibid.

201 Takemura Y, et al. The protective effect of good physical fitness when young on the risk of impaired glucose tolerance when old. *Prev Med.* 1999;28(1):14-19.

202 DiPietro L, et al. Moderate-intensity aerobic training improves glucose tolerance in aging independent of abdominal adiposity. *J Am Geriatr Soc.* 1998;46(7):875-879.

203 Ibid.

204 Henriksson J. Influence of exercise on insulin sensitivity. *J. Cardiovasc. Risk.* 1995; 4:303-309.

205 Walberg JL, et al. Exercise capacity and nitrogen loss during a high or Low-Carbohydrate diet. *Med Sci Sports Exerc.* 1988;20(1):34-43.

206 Langfort J, et al. Effect of Low-Carbohydrate-ketogenic diet on metabolic and hormonal responses to graded exercise in men *J Physiol Pharmacol.* 1996;47(2):361-371.

207 DiPasquale, M. High fat, high protein, Low-Carbohydrate diet: part I. *Drugs in Sports.* 1992;1(4):8-9.

208 Paffenbarger, RS, et al. Physical activity, other life-style patterns, cardiovascular disease and longevity. *Acta Med Scan.* 1986;711(suppl):85-91.

209 Paffenbarger, RS, et al. The association of changes in physical-activity and other lifestyle characteristics with mortality. *N Engl J Med.* 1993;328(8):538-545.

210 Vollmers S. The nineties fountain of youth. *Healthsport Newsletter.* 1999;7(3):3.